STAYING YOUNG

How to Look Good, Feel Better and Live Longer

STAYING YOUNG

How to Look Good, Feel Better and Live Longer

by

Frances Sheridan Goulart

PRENTICE-HALL, INC

Englewood Cliffs, N.J.

Prentice-Hall International, Inc., *London*
Prentice-Hall of Australia, Pty. Ltd., *Sydney*
Prentice-Hall Canada, Inc., *Toronto*
Prentice-Hall of India Private Ltd., *New Delhi*
Prentice-Hall of Japan, Inc., *Tokyo*
Prentice-Hall of Southeast Asia Pte. Ltd., *Singapore*
Editoria Prentice-Hall do Brasil Ltda., *Rio de Janeiro*
Prentice-Hall Hispanoamericana, S.A., *Mexico*

© 1987 by

Frances Sheridan Goulart

10 9 8 7 6 5 4 3 2 1

Library of Congress Cataloging-in-Publication Data

Goulart, Frances Sheridan.
  Staying young.

  Includes index.
  1. Longevity. 2. Nutrition. 3. Exercise.
4. Health. I. Title.
RA776.75.G68 1987   613   87-11369

ISBN 0-13-846213-5

ISBN 0-13-846205-4 {PBK}

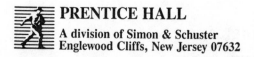 **PRENTICE HALL**
A division of Simon & Schuster
Englewood Cliffs, New Jersey 07632

Printed in the United States of America

DEDICATION

To my #1 worker bees, Esme O'Brien Carroll and Ivy Fischer Stone, and my loved ones at home: Ron, Sean-Lucien and Steffan Eamon

TABLE OF CONTENTS

STAYING YOUNG

How to Look Good, Feel Better and Live Longer

1

Staying Young: What You Can Do to Achieve It Starting Today

From King David who is said to have wooed young virgins in the hope of absorbing their vitality to the modern-day enthusiast for fetal lamb cell injections and vitamin E megadoses, people have been trying to stay younger longer.

Now medical researchers are growing more helpful. They say that medical advances and new insight into aging in recent years point to real progress on several fronts against mankind's most unrelenting enemy: time. Many, if not most of the biological hallmarks of age can, indeed, be delayed. You can reasonably expect to enjoy increased and sustained vitality after 30 if you know what habits save you from the rocking chair.

Data demonstrate that the average life span—that is, life expectancy—has been significantly extended, and there is every reason to suppose that it will continue to be as premature deaths from chronic ailments like heart disease, stroke and some cancers are prevented. In 1983, there were 32,000 Americans who were centenarians (people who have reached the age of 100 or better). In 1982, 2,890 centenarians were between the ages of 105 and 112.

Experts predict further that a century from today, the average American woman will live to be 90, with the average male doing almost as well. It seems possible that the maximum life span—that is, the longest that a human being can live—will be extended, too, from the present limit of about 115 years to as many as 140 happy, healthy years, conceivable only

1

if you are willing to forego the excesses of modern affluence and adhere to dietary limitations and other changes in living habits that this book explores in detail.

Researchers have discovered that some of the biological and mental declines characteristic of growing old are actually disease processes, not inevitable consequences of slowing down, and most of these changes-for-the-worst you can prevent.

"We used to think that all biological functions declined with age," noted Dr. Edward L. Schneider, deputy director of the National Institutes on Aging. "Now we know that certain important physiological processes stay the same, such as the output of the heart under stress and intelligence . . . Problems like arthritis, osteoporosis and senile dementia are really diseases that can be eliminated through various known and yet-to-be-discovered methods of prevention and treatment," says Schneider. For example, osteoporosis—the weakening of bones with age that is a leading killer and crippler of elderly Americans, especially women—is preventable by increasing calcium in your diet and staying physically active throughout life.

Dieting is one of the best tactics for a lengthier life and a leaner figure. Studies since the 1950's have shown that a prudent diet promotes longevity in animals by retarding the effects of aging on such important functions as immunity. In fact, "The only experimentally verified method of increasing the life expectancy of laboratory rats is restriction of calories," reported Dr. Michael McGinnis, director of the U. S. Office of Disease Prevention and Health Promotion.

Dr. Roy Walford, a pioneer in the study of aging and nutrition at the University of California at Los Angeles, had extensively compared the immune system of freely fed and diet-restricted mice and concluded that diet restriction contributes to a "younger" immune system.

A healthy immune system distinguishes foreign cells, such as germs and toxins, from the body's own cells and attacks the invaders. With advancing age, Walford reports, the immune system loses 10 to 20 percent of its ability to fight off invaders and it also becomes less adept at distinguishing "self" from "non-self" cells. Consequently, aging typically involves weakened defenses and "auto-immune" reactions in which the immune system mistakenly attacks the body's own tissues.

Dieting is one of the ways you can prevent this process. "Dietary restriction counteracts both the above trends," says Walford. Restriction of food intake can greatly retard the normal age-associated loss in certain cell receptors in the brain and extend your life by 40 percent.

Two human populations demonstrate this diet-longevity principle:

• In Okinawa, Japan, a small community that sticks to a "high-quality," low-calorie diet, including occasional fasting, has half of the aging-related diseases as the rest of the country.

• In Madrid, Spain, when the director of a nursing home, Dr. E. A.

Vallejo, placed half the in-patients on a diet alternating 2,300 calories one day with 800 calories the next day, in three years, the diet-restricted patients experienced half the incidence of death and half the frequency of infirmary admissions as the other patients.

This book will tell you how to put this reduced-caloric principle to work in your live-longer, live-better day.

Besides lowering calories, reduced salt and sugar, fewer fats and healthier food choices in general help. Excessive salt intake is directly related to the incidence of high blood pressure after 30 in the United States. Harold Battarbee, Ph.D., a noted hypertension researcher at Louisiana State University Medical Center, says Americans eat from 6 to 18 grams of salt a day—about three to nine scant teaspoons. But for optimum health—2 to 3 grams (one teaspoon a day) or less is better. What significance does this hold in holding back the aging process? "In populations where salt intake is less than 3 grams, we have found 70-year-olds with the blood pressure of 20-year-olds," says Dr. Battarbee.

Less sugar, besides increasing your energy and normalizing your weight, and improving your dental health, can also save you from disorders that are common in midlife. An epidemiological survey covering 21 countries recently reviewed by researchers at the University of Manchester (England) Medical School indicate that sucrose, more than fat, correlates with breast-cancer mortality in women over 30. (Younger breast-cancer victims don't show significant dietary tie-ins.) The link, they found, may be insulin, which "is an absolute requirement for the proliferation of normal mammary tissue, and 70 percent of experimental tumors may regress after destruction of the insulin-secreting capacity of the pancreas . . ." Okinawans, for example, have the lowest intake of sugar among the peoples of Japan; they also have the highest rate of centenarians and the greatest prevalence of healthy old people.

Ways to turn back the clock beginning with mealtime are detailed in this book—based on common-sense ideas that you are already familiar with: eat less fat, especially of the saturated type found in meat and dairy products; fewer cholesterol-containing and raising foods such as meats; more complex carbohydrates, such as whole-grain cereals, beans, vegetables, fruits and nuts; more fiber; more cruciferous vegetables and foods containing vitamins A and C, such as cabbage, broccoli, Brussels sprouts, carrots, tomatoes, oranges, leafy greens and winter squash and avoidance of refined starches and sugars and salt-cured, smoked or fried foods.

According to Richard S. Rivin, M.D., a professor of medicine and Chief of Nutrition at Memorial Sloan-Kettering Cancer Center and New York Hospital/Cornell Medical Center, "These changes can be expected to provide some cardiovascular and anti-cancer benefits, as well as improvement of obesity and diabetes."

Exercise is the next factor in feeling better after 30. According to Walter M. Bortz, M.D., of the Palo Alto Medical Clinic in California, "You can be old at 50 or young at 90 . . . If you go through a medical textbook and write down the things that happen with aging and then go to an exercise book and write down the things that result from inactivity, you'll find you've just about written the same things side by side." Physical activity can cut the rate of aging significantly and much more.

"More sedentary persons after 30 yearly lose about 1% of their capacity to work or exercise, and 50% of that loss is a result of inactivity," say experts. With exercise, that loss can be substantially regained.

A lack of fitness shows up throughout your body: decrease in heart function, flexibility, bone mass, muscular strength and mass, as well as the ability to take in and use oxygen. And it's the use of oxygen, which we know better as our "aerobic power" that's the biggest indicator of physical fitness. The scientific term is maximum volume of oxygen, or VO_2 max for short. VO_2 max is the all-important measure of how well you extract oxygen from the atmosphere, move it through your body channels and use it as energy. It relates intimately to all body functions.

Aerobic (oxygen-using) training, such as walking rapidly, swimming, rowing, jogging, square dancing or bicycling on a regular basis—no less than 30 minutes three times a week—can improve your VO_2 max, help return your weight to what it was at 25, keep your appetite down and your youthful spirits up. There's a plan in this book for you—for whatever your present level of fitness is now.

Consider one study of women swimmers, ages 70 and 71, measured against sedentary women the same age and athletic women in their early 20s. The older athletes had considerably less body fat than the sedentary women in their 70s and were well within the body-fat range of the 20-year-old active women. Their VO_2 max values were approximately twice those for normal women in their 70s and comparable to considerably younger non-athletes.

Another study, in groups of older men, found that VO_2 max declines at a "markedly retarded rate" in moderately active and athletic men. "If an inactive 70-year-old were to begin an exercise program at the level of moderate activity, the result would be a gain of 15 years in VO_2 max measurement," Dr. Bortz reported to the American Geriatrics Society. "If, however, the inactive subject were to achieve the athletic level of conditioning, there would be a potential improvement of 40 years. Exercise is the *single* most important ingredient in the elixir of youth," says Bortz.

And then there are food supplements that help you hold the line on aging. Do you really need them? Not if you don't mind turning into a 5 × 5 while you're meeting your needs. According to Philip Garry, Ph.D., director of the Clinical Nutrition Laboratory, University of New Mexico of Medicine, it would take 1,454 calories a day or 10,178 calories a week just to satisfy your body's minimum daily requirements if you skipped supplements.

How much is that in groceries a week? Loosen your belt. The list is 23 foods long and it runs from 4 tablespoons of salad oil to 6 ounces of round steak, 12 ounces of halibut and 9 ounces of salmon washed down with 1,227 calories worth of whole milk (eight glasses).

Don't think being well beyond your growth spurt years gets you off the hook. According to psychologist Mark McKinney, Ph.D., at the Department of Stress Medicine, University of Nebraska Center at Omaha, even a 95-pound woman of 40 has the same one-a-day needs as a 130-pound teenager because each one has roughly the same amount of bone to build and nerve endings to maintain. More, in fact.

What does change your nutrient needs are bad habits. Smoking and stress increase your vitamin C needs by 40 percent because with every passing decade your body absorbs vitamins and minerals less efficiently. According to biochemistry authority Dr. Lendon H. Smith, the anti-fatigue nutrient B-12 is often present in body tissues after 40 without being utilized while memory problems, common after 40, are a tipoff your B-6 needs are not being satisfied.

In short, living longer is a lot likelier if you add supplements to your life-extension diet and exercise plan. Exactly what and how much is discussed in the nutrients and supplements section (Pages 121–157).

As for breakthrough stuff? There's plenty of that, but if you can't get it without a prescription—it probably isn't good for you. Cellular therapy injections and chick embryo rejuvenation cocktails used at youth spas such as La Prairie in Switzerland and The Renaissance in the Bahamas, for example, are available only from doctors and must be used under close medical supervision. Gerovital GH3 (procaine), the so-called "youth pill" which is produced in the U.S. by Rom-Amer Pharmaceuticals of Las Vegas in joint venture with the government of Romania, where it was created, is another case in point. According to Dr. Norman Orenthreich, Clinical Associate professor of dermatology, N.Y.U. School of Medicine, and director of the Orenthreich Foundation for the Advancement of Science, "There is no evidence that procaine halts aging or has any powers of rejuvenation. The Gerovital data is totally unsupported and the product is nothing more than a much-touted panacea—with a questionable safety record . . . People have suffered allergic reactions to procaine, and in rare cases, it caused death from anaphylactic shock . . ."

If it's not safe, it's best left out of your live-longer day.

This book offers you a plan of action for eating, exercising and supplementing, plus pleasurable alternatives to your bad habits—including nicotine, alcohol or caffeine. Beat just one of these and you'll add years to your life. The caffeine in two and a half to three cups of coffee a day, for example, concludes a 1985 study by researchers at Stanford University School of Medicine, is associated with a rise in three cardiovascular risk factors—total cholesterol, low-density lipoprotein (LDL) cholesterol, and apolipoprotein B concentrations if you are sedentary and middle-aged.

Last but not least, this book will tell you how even friendship and faith can keep you younger longer. According to researchers at the University of Goteborg in Sweden, not being a lonely-only improves the quality of life and quadruples your chances of living longer. "The association between social activities and mortality is strong, even when all other factors are taken into account, indicating that an active social life . . . (is a) protection against premature death."

Best of all, an age-reduction program you follow for life can be fun. And to get you in the mood to have the time of your life from today on, here are a few amazing facts about aging:

• There are 32,000 people in the United States over 100—the women outnumber men. By the year 2020, the number of 100-plussers in the U.S. will increase by almost 200 percent (U.S. Census Bureau and Statistics from the Administration on Aging).

• Nuns live longer than women outside the church.

• Lobsters outlive all other shellfish but sea sponges have no known life span.

• Take up the test tube not the tuning fork: Chemists live three years longer than composers and military commanders (63 vs. 66).

• Reach out and touch someone: The death rate is twice as high for men and three times higher for women who have the fewest friends (UCLA Dr. Leslie Breslau, *New York Times*, October 2, 1984).

• Man's average life span has tripled since the days of the Roman gladiators (*Maximum Life Span*, W.W. Norton & Co).

• Small, smaller, smallest: Dwarfs live 200 years. Hobbits which are smaller live 100 years and gnomes, smallest of folklore's wee humans, live 400 years.

• New York State has the smallest 65-plus population in the U.S. Florida has the largest.

• The older you get the less sensitive to pain you become.

• Going, going, gone: The four diseases that keep most 85-year-olds from making it to 100 are heart disease, vascular disease, cancer and respiratory disorders.

• Don't dig, drink or dish the dirt: Next to coal miners—waiters, bartenders and newspaper reporters have the shortest life expectancy.

• Immanual Kant wrote his best philosophical works at 74 (*Guinness Book of World Records*).

• The older you get the fewer colds you get (*New York Times*, October 2, 1974).

• Long live art: The three professions in which men and women do their best work after 40 are musical comedy, novel writing and architecture (*The Average American Book*, NAL, 1980).

• A ball-point pen with black ink will last one year; those with blue ink, two years.

• One out of five married women has an extra-marital affair after 45.

- Male muscle hustle drops 10 percent every 10 years of age after the age of 20. At 60, a man has lost 60 percent of the capacity for exercise he had at 20.
- Smarter people live longer (*Curious Facts*, Holt, Rinehart, 1974).
- Short people have a life span 10 to 15 percent longer than that of taller people. America's five presidents who were less than 5'8" lived 80.2 years. Longevity for 6'1" and over averaged 66.6.
- Vitamins have life spans of three years—vitamin E a little longer, vitamin C a little shorter. Natural vitamins have the same life spans as synthetic.
- Peak ages for age-old ills: Heart attacks (45 and up); arthritis, rheumatism and diabetes (65 and up); high blood pressure (65 to 74); lung, colon, rectum, pancreas, stomach, ovaries, breast cancers (35 to 54); prostate, breast, uterus, stomach, colon and rectum (55 and up) (Gerontology Research Center in Maryland and the National Heart Institute).
- A $1 bill lasts about 18 months in circulation or for about 4,000 folds.
- Every year of involuntary unemployment reduces your life span by five years.
- The U.S. rates seventh as a longevity site (75 years average) preceded by Switzerland, Japan, Iceland, Sweden, Netherlands, Norway. Lowest life expectancy in the world—36 years—is in Afghanistan and West Africa (U.S. Census Bureau).
- Your chances of living longer are better if you live in Colorado rather than California.
- The brain of a 60-year-old uses the same amount of energy as a 10-watt light bulb.
- Have a happy day: Dissatisfaction with life increases your risk of premature death by at least 10 percent (Holistic Health Federation).
- Long in the foot: Good quality shoes can be expected to last three years in regular use (*Fascinating Facts*, Alfred Books, 1981).
- Skilled workers earn the most between 45–55. Big buck years for the unskilled is 20–30.
- Old and arty: Voltaire wrote *Candide* at age 64 and Will Durant finished his five-volume *History of Civilization* at age 89.
- A woman's capacity to exercise drops only 2 percent with each decade after 20. A trained woman can exercise up to 90 percent as vigorously at 60 as she could at 20.
- The average shoe worn by the average runner on an average surface lasts an average of 350 to 500 miles (Footwear Institute of America).
- Cancer is responsible for 12 percent of all deaths after 80; 30 percent of fatalities beween 65–69.
- Your sense of taste and smell declines 40–50% by age 60.
- During the average lifetime you burn 90 million calories per each pound of body weight.

- Army soap has a life span of five years in storage.
- Alzheimer's Disease (senile dementia) currently kills 100,000 40-plus Americans a year (National Institute of Health).
- One out of every five American males suffers a heart attack before the age of 55.
- A hard pencil will last for 30 miles of writing (30,000 words).
- "A better breakfast lengthens life," says University of California gerontologist Dr. Roy Walford. Walford's first meal of the day: 1 tablespoon brewer's yeast in low-sodium tomato juice, ⅔ cup rye cereal with wheat germ, fresh fruit and skim milk (*Maximum Life Span*, W. W. Norton & Co.).
- By the time you are 74, you will have eaten the combined weight of six elephants (*Boyd's Book of Odd Facts*).
- Going, going, gone: At 65 a man's muscle power is equal to that of a 25-year-old woman (Physical Fitness Institute).
- Nine out of 10 Americans over 35 have periodontal gum disease.
- Your body reaches its biological best at 26 (*Maximum Life Span*, W. W. Norton & Co.).

WHAT'S YOUR POTENTIAL FOR STAYING YOUNG? FIVE DO-IT-YOURSELF TESTS

"It's against my religion to talk about aging. I've got more energy than a lot of chorus girls. I'm just reaching my prime," observes plus-50 superstar Carol Channing.

Are you reaching yours? Or have you passed it prematurely? Are you in mentally and spiritually good shape; is your heart hearty and your lifestyle generally healthy?

Tip-top health that stands the test of time requires a sensible day-to-day diet, a lifestyle in which the good habits outnumber the bad, an optimistic outlook on life and an ability to tolerate stress.

Have you got what it takes? The following tests—based on criteria used by the American College of Physicians, American Cancer Society, American Heart Association and American Psychologists Association—will tell you how mentally and physically fit you are and how long you can expect to stay that way. Then do your homework to improve that potential by following the suggestions and plans that follow:

Test #1—How Young Is Your Body?

You know your chronological age in years, but what about your biological age? Here's a tailor-made test to tell you.

• *Aging Factors*	*Add*
Blood pressure 160/100 or over[1]	2 years
Overweight by 10 or more pounds	3 years
Cholesterol level higher than 250 mg.[1]	1 year
Smoker: more than half pack per day	2 years

- *Aging Factors*   *Add*

Drinker: more than 2 drinks per day	½ year
Poor post-exercise recovery (panting, shortness of breath, rapid heartbeat, muscular discomfort for more than a few hours)	1 year
Frequent chronic fatigue; anemia[1]	1 year
Poor immunity to infection (frequent colds or flu; infections of eye, ear, nose, throat; recurrent bladder or kidney infections)	1 year
Frequent constipation or diarrhea	1 year
Resting pulse rate over 80 beats per minute	½ year
Poor short-term memory (Do you forget where you left your glasses? Where you parked the car? Difficulty in recalling dates, appointments, names?)	1 year
Vision problems (short or farsightedness, astigmatism, do you have bifocals?)	½ year
Sexual difficulties or sexual apathy	½ year
If you have a history of chronic illnesses (allergy, bronchitis, ulcers, diabetes, etc.)	1 year

- *Anti-Aging Factors*   *Subtract*

Blood pressure 140/90 or under[1]	2 years
Cholesterol under 180[1]	1 year
No history of chronic illness (see above)	2 years
No asthma, allergies or respiratory troubles	1 year
Resting pulse rate 60 beats per minute or less	1 year
Good vision (don't wear glasses or use only for reading)	1 year

- *Scoring*

  - Start with your present age. Add or subract the years indicated according to which and what applies to you.[2] Total it up to arrive at your biological or true "body age." Refer to chapters in the book where you need improvements—diet, better meal planning, exercise, etc.

---

(1) Unless you've seen a doctor in the last six months, you'll need his help here.

(2) *Women Only*: Do you have osteoporosis, the post-menopause brittle bone disorder? Your doctor can order either a single energy CAT scan or dual photon absorptiometry test to check for spinal weakness that is a tip-off. Based on the readings, your doctor can calculate total bone mineral composition and determine the health of your skeleton, and prescribe the calcium you need to remedy things. Cost runs about $150 to $400.

Test #2—How Young Is Your Heart?

A healthy heart is found in a youthful body. If you've got one you've got the other. In fact, the health of your heart may be the factor that best determines how long and how well you'll hang in there, suggests both the International Heart Foundation and the American Heart Association. Here's a good way to test it out:

1. *Your Age.* Getting older increases everyone's chance of suffering heart disease. Anyone over 55 is likelier to have a heart attack or a stroke than a younger person. There is nothing you can do but consider this factor and count it in.
   - If you are 56 or over—score 1.
   - If you are 55 or younger—score 0.

2. *Sex.* Men are at a greater risk of cardiovascular complication than women (the occurrence of heart attacks among women is increasing though).
   - If you are male—score 1.
   - If you are female—score 0.

3. *Family History.* If you come from a family where there is or has been cardiovascular disease your chances of being a victim, too, rise—especially if one or more of your close relatives—grandparents, parents, brothers or sisters—suffered an attack or stroke before age 60.
   - For one or more close blood relatives who have had a heart attack or stroke at or before the age of 60—score 12.
   - For one or more close blood relatives with a known history of heart disease at or before age 60 but no heart attacks or strokes—score 10.
   - For one or more who have had a heart attack or stroke after the age of 60—score 6.
   - Otherwise—score 0.

4. *Personal History.* If you, yourself, have a history of cardiovascular disease, your chances of more trouble are greater than a non-victim's.
   - If you have had one or more at or before the age of 50: a heart attack, heart or blood vessel surgery or a stroke—score 20.
   - If you have had one or more after the age of 50—score 10.
   - If you have had none—score 0.

5. *Diabetes.* Cardiovascular disease runs high among diabetics. If you are a diabetic, check the statement below that applies:
   - If you had diabetes before age 40 and are now on insulin—score 10.
   - If you had diabetes at or before age 40 and are now on insulin or pills—score 5.
   - If your diabetes is controlled by diet, or your diabetes began after age 55—score 3.

- If you have never had diabetes—then make your score 0.

6. *Smoking.* Carbon monoxide in the bloodstream competes with oxygen for transport to the cells in the body, reducing the amount of oxygen available for use in your body's cells. To counteract this effect, your heart must work harder supplying oxygen to all cells. CO damages the lining of the arterial blood vessels and increases deposit of materials that lead to atherosclerosis. Smoking also causes blood vessels to narrow. This is a risky condition called vasoconstriction.

- If you smoke two or more packs of cigarettes a day—score 10.
- If you smoke between one and two packs a day or quit smoking less than a year ago—score 6.
- If you smoke 6 or more cigars a day or a pipe regularly—score 6.
- If you smoke less than one pack of cigarettes a day or quit smoking more than a year ago—score 3.
- If you smoke less than 6 cigars a day or do not inhale a pipe regularly—score 3.
- If you have never smoked—score 0.

7. *Diet.* A diet rich in cholesterol and saturated fat gives you a greater risk of heart disease. High cholesterol and triglyceride (other fatty material) levels in the blood cause atherosclerotic deposits in the lining of the arteries. As the deposits build, arteries narrow and the flow is slowed.

- In your regular eating pattern if you have at least one serving of red meat daily, more than seven eggs a week, use butter, whole milk, and cheese daily—score 8.
- In your regular eating pattern if you eat red meat four to six times a week, eat four to seven eggs a week, use margarine, low-fat dairy products and some cheese—score 4.
- If you eat poultry, fish and a little or no red meat, three or fewer eggs a week, some margarine, skim milk, and skim milk products—score 0.

8. *Cholesterol.*

- If your cholesterol level is 276 or above—score 10.
- If it is between 225 and 275—score 5.
- If it is 224 or below—score 0.

9. *High Blood Pressure.* When blood pressure goes above normal range and stays there you have hypertension—meaning your heart must pump harder to get blood through arterial passages. When blood pressure is normal, chances of heart trouble are lower.

- If either number in your blood pressure reading is 160 over 100 (160/100) or higher—score 10.
- If either number is 140 over 90 (140/90) but less than 160 over 100 (160/100)—score 5.
- If both numbers are less than 140 over 90 (140/90)—score 0.

10. *Weight.* The heavier you are, the more you tip the scales in favor of a heart attack. Is your weight up, down or on the nose?

• Your height, ____ feet ____ inches, minus 5 feet = ____ inches over 5 feet.

• Multiply inches over 5 feet, ____ by 5 pounds = ____ pounds per inch over 5 feet.

• Add pounds per inch over 5 feet, ____, plus 110 pounds (men) or 100 pounds (women) = ____ pounds, ideal weight.

• Subtract your ideal weight, ____ pounds, from your present weight, ____ pounds, = ____ pounds overweight.

• If you are at least 25 pounds overweight—score 4.

• If you are 10 to 24 pounds overweight—score 2.

• If you are less than 10 pounds overweight—score 0.

11. *Exercise.* Physical activity is essential. A lack aggravates heart problems.

• If you engage in any aerobic exercise (brisk walking, jogging, bicycle, racquetball, swimming) for more than 15 minutes less than once a week—score 4.

• If you exercise that hard once or twice a week—score 2.

• If you engage in that exercise three or more times a week—score 0.

12. *Stress.* Certain personality types are more prone to cardiovascular disorders than others. If you are a hurried, harried type who never finds time to enjoy life in the slow lane, you are a more likely candidate for a heart condition.

• If you are frustrated when waiting in line, often in a hurry to complete work or keep appointments, easily angered, irritable—score 4.

• If you are simply impatient when waiting, occasionally hurried, or occasionally moody—score 2.

• If you are relatively comfortable when waiting, seldom rushed, and easygoing—score 0.

Scoring:

To get a total, check it against the chart below. A high score does not mean you will develop heart disease as you age, but that there's a potential risk.

High risk* .... 40 and above.
Medium risk 20–39
Low risk .... 19 and below.

---

*Based on a consideration of your risk factors, and if need be, other more sophisticated testing, a professional heart clinic can thoroughly rate your risk if it's high and prescribe measures to help you avoid becoming part of the grim statistics. Call your local heart association chapter office for details.

Test #3—Rate Your Fitness

There are plenty of ways to measure fitness but what's one standard against which you can best measure your fitness? Yourself.

Based on evaluations and standards set by the National Heart Institute, President's Council on Physical Fitness and the Aerobics Institute of America, the following test does it best because you do it twice. Take it today, then repeat the 10 physical activities routine in three months. It's the only way to get a clear picture of your progress toward your fitness goals and your potential. The tests below measure aerobic ability, flexibility, strength, balance, coordination, relaxation and concentration. Be sure to warm up and stretch before. Omit any test that might cause undue stress.

Instructions and scoring

Get a partner to help with details and timing. Enter the date of the first test at the top of the first column with the results below. Enter the second set of results three months later in column 2. Score 5 points for each activity in which you improve and minus 5 in each activity you don't. Score 0 if there is no change. Total it up.

1. *12-minute run/jog/walk*: Select a level course of known length. The gym or running track at the Y is ideal. See how far you can travel on foot in 12 minutes. If you can't run the whole way, jog. If you can't jog, walk. Don't strain yourself; walking the whole way is fine. Hint: beginners almost invariably start out too fast. Enter your distance. (Aerobics)

2. *Sitting toe-reach*: Sit with the base of your spine firmly against a wall or other supporting structure. Extend your legs straight out in front of you just far enough apart so that both hands, palms down, can fit between your knees. Do not bend your knees. Gently reach forward, sliding your hands along the floor. Be sure to keep the base of your spine against the wall. Reach as far as you can and hold the position for five seconds. Your partner marks that point, then measures its distance from the wall. Enter that distance. (Flexibility)

3. *Prone chin-lift*: Lie facedown with your hands along your sides. Raise your head as high as you can and hold it for 5 seconds. Have your partner measure the distance between your chin and the surface on which you are lying. Enter the distance. (Flexibility, strength)

4. *Standing long jump*: Stand with your feet together, toes just behind a line. Keeping the feet next to each other, see how far you can jump forward. Your partner measures the length of the jump. Make three jumps. Enter the best distance at right. (Strength, power, concentration)

5. *Jump and reach*: With your feet flat on the ground, reach up with one hand and touch a wall as high as you can without stretching. Your partner marks that spot. Then jump straight up to touch the wall as high as you can. Your partner marks the second spot. Lastly, measure the distance

between the two. Make three jumps and enter the best distance. (Strength, power, concentration)

6. *Flexed-arm hang*: Use a chinning bar or the equivalent for this test. Skip this if you have not practiced chinning or other upper body exercises in recent years. With your palms toward your face, grasp the bar. Use something to stand on or have your partner help you get high enough so that your eyes are level with the bar. Hang at that level as long as you can while your partner times you. Enter the time. (Strength, concentration)

7. *One-foot blind balance*: On a firm, level surface, stand on one foot with eyes closed for as long as you can without shifting the supporting foot or touching the ground with the other foot. Do this three times while your partner times you. Enter the best time. (Balance)

8. *Shuttle run*: On a level surface, place two markers (any clearly visible objects will do) 10 yards apart. Stand behind the first marker. Go around it as fast as you can. Come back to the first marker, around it to the second marker again, then back to the first marker to finish. Your partner times these two round trips. Take the best time of three tries and enter it. (Strength, power, coordination, balance, concentration)

9. *Wastebasket toss*: Stand exactly 9 feet from a wastebasket. Using an underhand toss, try to throw a small ball into the basket. The size of the ball and basket is unimportant, as long as the two are the same in both tests. Toss the ball 20 times and count the number of times you get the ball in the basket. Try the 20 tosses three times. Enter the best score. (Coordination, concentration)

10. *Horizontal arm extension*: Extend both arms in front of you. See how long you can keep them horizontal. Your partner should not offer encouragement, but should simply end the test whenever either arm drops more than 1 inch below horizontal. Enter the time. (Relaxation, strength, concentration)

Analyzing your score

40 to 50: Superb

30 to 40: Excellent

20 to 30: Good

15 to 20: Fair

Test #4—How Healthy Is Your Diet?

Eating enough is easy. We spend an hour and 30 minutes a day doing nothing but. Eating enough of the right stuff three times a day is something else again. Surveys tell us more than 36 percent of us skip breakfast and 90 percent of us snack at least once a day, if not more.

A poor diet results in nutrient deficiencies which raises the risk of heart disease, lowered immune function, diabetes and more. To health rate *your* diet, answer the following questions, keep track of the pluses and minuses you accumulate, then subtract the latter from the former to get your total.

Scoring

51 to 88: Excellent

21 to 50: Good. You've a diet to be proud of. Keep it up.

10 to 20: You need help.

1. How many fast-food meals do you have a week? (Salad bar snacks don't count.)
Answers: a) none; b) 1; c) 2; d) 3; e) 4 or more
Score: a) +3; b) 0; c) −1; d) −2; e) −3.

2. How often do you drink? (One serving = 12 oz. regular or light beer, 4 oz. wine, 1 oz. liquor.)
Answers: a) 1 or less a week; b) 2–3 a week; c) 4–6 a week; d) 1–2 a day; e) more than 2 a day
Score: a) +3; b) +1; c) −1; d) −2; e) −3.

3. How many of your weekly meals include cheese? (Low fat cottage cheese doesn't count; cream cheese snacks, pizza, cheeseburgers, cheese and meat dishes do.)
Answers: a) 1 or less; b) 2–3; c) 4–5; d) 6 or more
Score: a) +2; b) +1; c) −2; d) −3.

4. How often do you have fish or shellfish (other than deep-fried entrees or fishsticks)?
Answers: a) none; b) 1–2; c) 3–4; d) 5 or more
Score: a) −2; b) +1; c) +2; d) +3.

5. How often do you eat deep-fried foods in any four-week period (fish, chicken, vegetables, snack foods)?
Answers: a) none; b) 1–2; c) 3–4; d) 5 or more
Score: a) +3; b) 0; c) −1; d) −3.

6. How often a week are cold cuts or other processed meats (franks, bacon, sausage) on the menu?
Answers: a) none; b) 1–2; c)3–4; d) 5 or more
Score: a) +3; b) +2; c) −1; d) −3.

7. How often per week do you eat freshly prepared red meat (steak, roast beef, beef patties, lamb, pork chops, etc.)?
Answers: a) 1 or less; b) 2–3; c)4–5; d) 6 or more
Score: a) +3; b) +2; c) −1; d) −3.

8. How many times a day do you have vegetables? (One serving = ½ cup; potatoes count.)
Answers: a) none; b) 1; c)2; d) 3; e) 4 or more
Score: a) −3; b) 0; c) +1; d) +2; e) +3.

9. How many servings do you eat of the cancer-proofing cruciferous vegetables (broccoli, cauliflower, cabbage, Brussels sprouts, greens, kale, kohlrabi, turnips)?

Answers: a) none; b) 1–3; c) 4–6; d) 7 or more

Score: a) −3; b) +1; c) +2; d) +3.

10. How many servings of fruits or vegetables do you eat a week to get vitamin A and beta-carotene (vegetable form of vitamin A)? (Carrots, pumpkins, sweet potatoes, cantaloupe, spinach, winter squash, greens, apricots, broccoli.)

Answers: a) none; b) 1–3; c) 4–6; d) 7 or more

Score: a) −3; b) +1; c) +2; d) +3.

11. Do you eat chicken and turkey without the skin?

Answers: a) yes; b) no; c) don't eat any

Score: a) +3; b) −3; c) +3.

12. What do you spread on bread, toast and muffins?

Answers: a) butter; b) cream cheese; c) margarine; d) diet margarine; e) jam; f) sugar-reduced spreads or nothing

Score: a) −3; b) −3; c) −2; d) −1; e) 0; f) +3.

13. What do you like to drink most?

Answers: a) fruit juices; b) water or club soda; c) diet soda; d) coffee or tea; e) soda or fruit drink

Score: a) +3; b) +3; c) −1; d) −1; e) −3.

14. How much caffeine do you drink daily? (1 serving = one cup coffee, 1 cup regular tea or 12 oz. regular cola.)

Answers: a) none; b) 1; c) 2; d) 3; e) 4 or more

Score: a) +3; b) +1; c) −1; d) −2; e) −3.

15. How do you usually season your meals?

Answers: a) garlic or lemon juice; b) herbs or spices; c) soy sauce; d) salt; e) nothing

Score: a) +3; b) +3; c) −2; d) −3; e) +3.

16. Which of these snacks do you eat most?

Answers: a) fruit or vegetables; b) pre-sweetened yogurt; c) salted nuts; d) chips; e) cookies; f) granola bar; g) candy bar

Score: a) +3; b) +2; c) −1; d) −2; e) −2; f) −2; g) −3.

17. Which breakfast would you pick?

Answers: a) croissant or doughnut; b) fried eggs and white toast; c) just coffee or nothing

Score: a) −3; b) −3; c) −2.

18. How many times do you have canned or made-from-a-mix soup a week? (Low-sodium and health brands don't count.)

Answers: a) none; b) 1–2; c) 3–4; d) 5 or more

Score: a) +3; b) 0; c) −2; d) −3.

19. How many egg yolks do you have weekly? (Include soufflés, omelets, egg puddings, etc.)

Answers: a) 2 or less; b) 3–4; c) 5–6; d) 7 or more
Score: a) +3; b) +2; c) −1; d) −3.

20. Which would you pick for dessert? (Don't include low-fat, sugar-free versions.)

Answers: a) pie or cake; b) ice cream; c) yogurt, ice milk or fruit ice; d) fresh fruit or no dessert
Score: a) −3; b) −3; c) +1; d) +3.

21. How many calcium-rich foods do you eat a day? (1 serving = ⅔ cup milk, yogurt; 1 oz. cheese; 1½ oz. sardines; 3 oz. salmon or 5 oz. tofu; 1 cup leafy greens or broccoli.)

Answers: a) none; b) 1; c) 2; d) 3 or more
Score: a) −3; b) +1; c) +2; d) +3.

22. What of these sandwich fillings would you choose?

Answers: a) meat; b) cheese; c) peanut butter; d) tuna, crab or salmon; e) chicken or turkey
Score: a) −3; b) −1; c) +1; d) +3; e) +3.

23. What else do you use in sandwiches?

Answers: a) mayonnaise; b) low-fat, low-salt mayonnaise; c) mustard or ketchup; d) nothing
Score: a) −2; b) −1; c) 0; d) +3.

24. Which of these "extras" do you eat at a salad bar?

Answers: a) nothing, lemon, vinegar; b) reduced-calorie dressing; c) regular dressings and/or croutons, bacon bits; d) cole slaw, pasta salad, potato salad
Score: a) +3; b) +1; c) −1; d) −1.

25. What type of milk do you use?

Answers: a) whole; b) 2% lowfat; c) 1% lowfat; d) ½% or skim; e) none
Score. a) −2; b) 0; c) +2; d) +3; e) 0.

26. Check the number of meals you have weekly that include dried beans, split peas or lentils?

Answers: a) none; b) 1; c) 2; d) 3 or more
Score: a) −1; b) +1; c) +2; d) +3.

27. How many whole-grain foods do you eat daily? (Sugar-coated cereal doesn't count; sugar-free cereals, whole-wheat pancakes, cooked cereal, brown or converted rice, bulgur (wheat), rye bread, etc. do.)

Answers: a) none; b) 1–2; c) 3–4; d) 5–6; e) 7 or more
Score: a) −3; b) 0; c) +1; d) +2; e) +3.

28. How many servings of fresh fruit or juice do you have a day? (One serving = 1 piece of fruit or 6 oz. juice.)

Answers: a) none; b) 1; c) 2; d) 3; e) 4 or more
Score: a) −3; b) 0; c) +1; d) +2; e) +3.

29. Do you eat lean meats only?

Answers: a) yes; b) no; c) don't eat meat at all
Score: a) +3; b) −3; c) +3.

30. What type of bread do you prefer?

Answers: a) whole wheat; b) rye; c) pumpernickel; d) white

Score: a) +3; b) +2; c) +2; d) −2.

Test #5—What's Your Preventive Medicine IQ?

Sometimes it pays to leave your doctoring to the doctor. Do you know when each of the following age-proofing medical tests should be done?

Check one

M = Monthly

Q = Quarterly (every three months)

S = Semi-annually (every six months)

A = Annually

Answers below. Score one for each correct answer.

1. Blood Pressure (heart/circulation)
2. Hearing Function
3. Reflex Testing (knee-jerks, wrist)
4. Sensory and Smell Function
5. Glucose (blood sugar)
6. Skin Observations and Skin (saltiness)
7. Urine Tests (a check on pH of urine as well as bilirubin, blood glucose, ketones, nitrite, protein and urobilinogen content)
8. Visual Acuity (eye and vision tests)
9. Hemoglobin (blood tests)
10. Feces Observations
11. Dizziness and Ataxia (nervous system tests)
12. Urea Nitrogen (blood tests)
13. Pulse Measurements (two-step exercise)
14. Dental Plaque Disclosure (your dentist does this)
15. Pulmonary Function Measurements for Forced Vital Capacity
16. Testicle Observations (men)
17. Hair Observations and Mineral Analysis
18. Mammogram (women)
19. A Tetanus and Polio Booster Shot
20. Pap Smear Test
21. Blood and Cholesterol
22. Stool Blood Test (for bowel cancer)
23. Complete Physical

Answers

Numbers 2, 4, 5, 12, 13, 17 are annual.

Numbers 3, 11 are semi-annually (every six months)

Numbers 8, 9, 10 are quarterly (every three months)
Numbers 1, 6, 7, 14, 15, 16 are monthly
18. Yearly after 40
19. Every five years
20. Every five years
21. Every two years after 30, yearly after 50
22. Every two years after 30, yearly after 50
23. Every one to three years

Scoring

23 to 18: Excellent

17 to 12: Good

11 or Less: Time to check in for a checkup

2

Natural Ingredients for Looking Good, Feeling Better and Living Longer

From a 30-plus point of view, all foods fall into one of two categories—the kind that set your body clock forward and the kind that set it back. You don't even need a guide to avoid category two. If it's high in fat, sugar, salt or chemical additives, or comes to you richly endowed with calories, it's got age-you-faster potential. This goes for all the foods in circles 1 and 2 of the Staying Young Ingredient Chart (Figure 2–1). But there's plenty left to make a meal out of in circles 3 and 4. Here are 25 foods that do the most to lead you astray and the ones that do the most to keep you on the straight and youthful narrow. Help yourself!

THE 25 FOODS THAT GIVE YOU THE GREATEST HEALTH BENEFITS

- *Nucleic Acids and Fermented Foods*
  - Everyday Foods That Help You Look 10 to 12 Years Younger
  - How Sauerkraut and Sourdough Prevent Colitis, Ulcers and Hemorrhoids
  - Are You Eating What the World's Healthiest Old People Eat?
  - The Magic of Nucleic Acid Foods
  - Beat the Flu and the Common Cold with Brewer's Yeast

21

THE STAYING YOUNG INGREDIENT TARGET

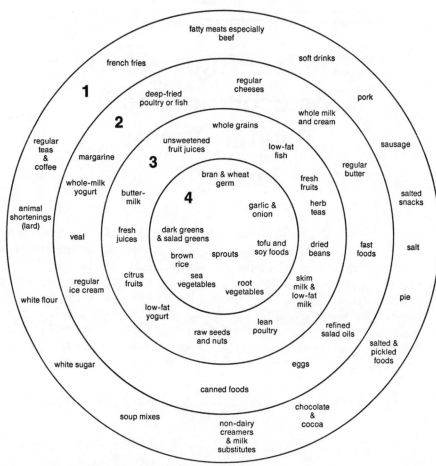

- Circles 3 and 4 contain the foods that are highest in vitamins, minerals and life-lengthening elements.
- Circle 2 are foods to use in moderation.
- Circle 1 are anti-aging foods to avoid.

Figure 2-1

- What the USDA says About the Special Benefits of Brewer's Yeast
- The #1 Way to Get More Chromium for Staying Young
- Do You Need a B-vitamin Brewer's Yeast Boost?
- Yeast: The World's Oldest Superfood
- How to Add Brewer's Yeast to Your Daily Meals
- Top Sources of Nucleic Acids and Fermented Foods
- Top Sources of Brewer's Yeast

- *Tropical, Citrus and Raw Fruits*
  - How Fruit Helps You Fight the 12 Most Common Signs of Aging
  - The Magic Fiber in Fruit Flushes Carcinogens from Your Body
  - A Low-Calorie Way to Lower Your Blood Pressure
  - Special Nutritional Benefits of Tropical Fruits
  - Reach for a Peach Instead of a Popsicle
  - Top Fruit Sources of Youth-Enhancing Nutrients

- *Yogurt, Acidophilus and Other Cultured Dairy Products*
  - Are You Eating the Foods of the Gods Everyday?
  - A Better-than-Milk Source of Age-Proofing Calcium
  - Women: Prevent Premature Aging with Breakfast!
  - Lower Your Cholesterol Level with Yogurt
  - Yogurt Helps Prevent Candida Infections
  - Yogurt—A Rare Source of the Essential Vitamin K
  - Yogurt Can Help You Unwind During the Day, Sleep Better at Night
  - Tips for Buying Yogurt
  - How Yogurt is Made
  - Yogurt Alternatives
  - Top Sources of Cultured Milks

- *Seaweeds and Sea Vegetables*
  - Revitalize Your Adrenal Glands with Salt Substitutes
  - A Weed with 100 Times the Blood-Building Iron of Spinach
  - Reduce Your Risk of Post-40 Diabetes; End Constipation and Hypoglycemia
  - Are You Using the World's Richest Source of B-12?

- *Root Vegetables*
  - Six All-Star Vegetables with the Best Artery-Cleansing Effect
  - The Nucleic Acid Staying Young Diet That Helps You Look and Feel Better in Two Weeks
  - What Cornell University Nutritionists Say About the Youth Factor in Potatoes
  - How Horseradish and Carrots Protect Your Heart and Vision
  - Best Root Vegetables for Staying Young

- *Garlic and Onions*
  - Use Onions to Reduce Inflammations, Allergic Reactions and Block Asthma
  - Sulphur—The Cancer-Blocking Trace Mineral in Onions and Garlic
  - Allicin—The Better-than-Drugs Remedy for High Cholesterol, Hypertension and Headaches
  - Fight 15 Infections with Onions
  - Top Sources of Garlic
  - Top Sources of Onions

- *Sprouted Grains, Beans and Herbs*
  - Why the National Heart and Diabetes Institute Puts Alfalfa on the Menu
  - Get More Vitamins and Minerals with Sprouts
  - Sprouts May Help Prevent Cancer
  - Put Zip in Your Life for Zero Calories
  - Sprouts—A Top Source of Fat-Free Protein
  - How to Grow Your Own Sprouts
  - Source of Age-Proof Sprouts

- *Honey, Pollen, Propolis*
  - Three Sweet-Tooth Foods That Help You Stay Young
  - Use Pollen as a Rejuvenator
  - Six Amazing Reasons Pollen Makes You Look and Feel Younger
  - Propolis—Nature's Wonder Drug
  - Seven Ways to Use Propolis Regularly
  - Do You Know What Famous First Family Uses Propolis Daily?
  - Honey—Keep it in Your Medicine Cabinet
  - Six Special Benefits Honey Supplies

- Honey vs. Sugar: Important Facts
- Tips on Shopping for Honey
- Top Sources of Bee Foods

"Old age," statesman Bernard Baruch once observed, "is 15 years younger than I am."

A Salad a Day . . .

One way to live longer? More life-extension cole slaws and Caesar salads. At 10 high-fiber calories a cup, leafy greens keep your calories down and cardiovascular health under control. For example, if you weigh 154 now at age 30, keep your exercise up but *don't* cut any calories, you'll weigh in at 200 by the time you're 60 and be a prime-of-life candidate for arteriosclerosis, to say nothing of losing self-esteem and becoming a less-than-attractive risk to your insurance company.

Unlike the no-fiber cheeseburgers you may be munching on now, a whole-meal midday salad is rich in roughage and low in sodium, the mineral that hikes hypertension. "In populations where salt intake is less than 3 grams we find 70-year-olds with the blood pressure of 20-year-olds," says fitness consultant Charles Kuntzleman. (A whole head of lettuce has less than 50 mg. of sodium; a triple cheeseburger hold the fries, has almost 2 grams of sodium.)

After grains and fruits, greens are the third best dietary source of fiber to control blood cholesterol and check diabetes. A quart of salad with low-fat dressing even has 75 percent less saturated fat than a Ritz cracker. You can't lose. (The only live-longer nutrients you *do* miss in any measurable amount are B complex and vitamin D. But a good egg and nut oil dressing even adds those.)

Ounce for ounce, leafy green meals also supply more potassium, fiber and vitamins A and C than meat, fish or fowl, go-together minerals zinc and iron, as well as trace minerals and antioxidants, and respectable amounts of calcium, too. One cup of spinach or beet greens—with only 1/10 the calories of cottage cheese—supplies almost 25 percent of a woman's daily need for this osteoporosis-preventing mineral.

University Studies Call Lettuce an Anti-Depressant and Sleep Aid

Lettuce even helps prevent post-30's depression and promotes sleep. "Leafy green vegetables are one simple way to help prevent and overcome anemia caused by iron deficiency[1] which leads to lack of energy, fatigue, anxiety and insomnia," concludes a study by University of Wisconsin Nutritional and Food Science researchers. Twenty-five percent of the population over 35 shows a lower-than-it-ought-to-be intake of iron, an essen-

---

[1]After calcium, iron is the mineral found in the greatest amount in the body.

tial mineral that prevents headaches, intestinal malabsorption of foods, and keeps your ability to savor the flavor in foods keen.

A life filled with lettuce also supplies blood-enriching chlorophyll and the anti-blood-clotting factor vitamin K. Vitamin K, like calcium, helps prevent or remedy bone disorders including as much as 50 percent, according to the new Japanese nutrition research. Three A-1 sources of K? Common lettuce, spinach and turnip greens.

In fact, greens may prevent you from turning gray. The nutrients in greens improve your body's hormone balance, nutritional status and resistance to stress. And those are three out of the six factors (the other three are chemicals, disease and radiation) that researchers say cause hair color to fade.[2]

Why Skin Specialists Recommend Leafy Greens

Lettuce is good for lots of vitamin C, and according to California dermatologist Dr. Harry Daniell, "It is likely that relatively high doses of this antioxidant vitamin can help to slow down the aging process in general, including a retardation of skin wrinkling." Vitamin C is essential to the formation of the skin's collagen.

Lettuce is leafy green medicine for dry post-30's skin. Greens are 90 percent water making them nature's #1 aid in maintaining the proper acid-alkali mantle in the skin. The vitamin C in double-dip helpings of plain romaine or not-so-plain arugula can also help you save your teeth by "significantly decreasing your susceptibility to periodontal disease which afflicts nine out of ten post-35's," says Paul H. Keyes, D.D.S., researcher of the Nutritional Institute of Dental Research in Bethesda, Maryland.

A low-calorie leaf can even replace a slice of high-calorie bread: Sprinkle with sprouts or a spread and roll up, and you have a hand-held life-extension salad. Here's approximately what a quarter pound helping of eight good greens provide:

Greens	Vitamin A (I.U.)	Vitamin C (mg.)	Calcium (mg.)	Iron (mg.)	Potassium (mg.)
Crisphead lettuce (iceberg, great lakes)	375	7	23	0.6	199
Parsley, curly	9,640	195	230	7	825

---

[2]Hair color is determined by many factors, mainly the amount, type and distribution of the dark pigment called melanin. There are as many as 3,000 melanocytes for every square millimeter of skin; they transport melanin to hair follicles. Aging causes the melanocytes to slow or stop the production of melanin, separate from the hair follicles and interrupt or reduce the flow of melanin to the developing hair. Without melanin, the hair turns gray. Fill your bowl.

Greens	Vitamin A (I.U.)	Vitamin C (mg.)	Calcium (mg.)	Iron (mg.)	Potassium (mg.)
Spinach	9,185	58	106	3.5	533
Kale	11,340	211	282	3.1	429
Beet greens	6,918	34	135	3.8	647
Swiss chard	7,370	36	100	3.6	624
Looseleaf lettuce (oak leaf, ruby, black-seeded Simpson)	2,155	21	77	1.6	300
Buttercrunch or Boston	1,100	9	40	2.3	300

Source: USDA Handbook No. 8.

Best sources of leafy greens

- Amaranth[3]
- Arugula
- Bok Choy Cabbage
- Beet Greens and Swiss Chard
- Bibb
- Boston (buttercrunch)
- Broccoli Raab (rape)
- Butterhead Lettuces
- Cabbage (red and green)
- Celery Cabbage (Chinese cabbage, napa)
- Chicory
- Corn Salad (also called field lettuce or mache)
- Dandelion Greens
- Endive (curly-leaf)
- Belgian Endive (Witloof)
- Escarole (broad leaved endive, chickory escarole)
- Fiddlehead Fern (or crosiers), sold only in the spring
- Iceberg Lettuce
- Kale
- Mustard, Turnip and Collard Greens
- Oakleaf Lettuce

---

[3]See *Sources*.

- Radicchio
- Romaine (Cos lettuce)
- Sorrel (sour grass, dock)
- Spinach
- New Zealand Spinach
- Watercress and Garden Cress

HOW FRUIT HELPS YOU FIGHT THE 12 MOST COMMON SIGNS OF AGING

There is nothing better to put on your list of tricks of time-fighting foods than fruit. According to UNESCO reports, says Ronald E. Goss, director of the National Advisory Service in Washington, D.C., Pakistan's Hunzans are the only cancer-free people in the world, and what they eat is one of the reasons. Next to glacial water and yogurt, their favorite food is fruit.

Going bananas, apples or pears is a good idea for you, too, because out of 12 commonest signs of aging that include dry skin, thinning hair, periodontal disease, poor posture, varicose veins, elevated blood pressure, stiff joints and high cholesterol levels—fiber-rich fruit—especially tropical fruits—help prevent eight of them, says Dr. Richard Weindrich of UCLA Medical School.

The Magic Fiber in Fruit Flushes Carcinogens from Your Body

Fiber's the first reason, nutrients are the second and water content may be the third. Fruit is a first-rate source of a special fiber called pectin. All fibers soften the stool and improve the speed of bowel movements—which researchers say helps flush out cancer-causing toxins. But pectin does something more. "For some reason, a water-holding fiber like cellulose has no influence on serum cholesterol levels," says biochemist David Kritchevsky, Ph.D. "But water-soluble fibers like pectin can reduce cholesterol."

A Low-Calorie Way to Lower Your Blood Pressure

Most good fruits give you less than 100 calories a serving and with it generous amounts of age-fighting A, C, D, calcium and potassium. The higher your intake of potassium-rich fruits, says the National Health Systems Syndicate, the lower your blood pressure. And fruits can help you kick a candy bar habit. (Sweetest of the sweet? Pineapples, mangos, cherries, figs and bananas.)

A good fruit is even a two-for-one food providing water as well as solid nutrition (most fruits are 80%–90% water). New British studies indicate that many symptoms of senility can be alleviated by adding six or more dehydration-preventing glasses of fluid a day to your diet.

Special Nutritional Benefits of Tropical Fruits

And if you're allergic to oranges, don't have a doughnut for breakfast instead. Just switch your citrus or try a tropical fruit. Besides the bargain-basement calories (50 a serving), grapefruit (which originated in China where they're still served as an appetizer) are low in sodium, high in potassium and so versatile you can use them the way California's Coachella Valley grapefruit lovers do—in chili, in homemade mayonnaise or to marinate fish.

What the French call pampelmousse is even remedial. "The bitter tea of grapefruit," says herbalist Eloise Allison, "is as effective as quinine and has no side effects. It relieves the aches and discomfort associated with infectious diseases. Onions or garlic cooked with grapefruit make it doubly effective."

You don't need oranges to get your vitamin C. One non-citrus, high-C fruit with twice the C of oranges and half the calories (45) is the New Zealand emerald-green kiwi fruit which even Mom and Pop stores carry. Other uncommon fruits with more vitamin C than oranges, says the United Fruit and Vegetable Association, include the following (*starred entries are also rich in calcium or vitamin A or beta-carotene*): guava, cherimoya,* papaya,* prickly pear,* plantain, kumquats, passion fruit.

Reach for a Peach Instead of a Popsicle

Fresh fruits even make good ice cream bar alternatives. Here's a neat way to eat a juicy mango—a larger-than-life peach taste-alike with fewer calories than banana and five times more age-proof beta-carotene: Take a fork and push it into the fattest end of the mango, keeping the tines as close to the seeds as possible. Peel from the other end for a mango-on-a-stick dessert. You can't eat it all, but when you get to the fork, grasp the exposed seed, remove fork and munch on.

And don't pass up dried fruit to skimp on calories. One-half a cup of dried banana chips has as much vitamin A, potassium and phosphorus and seven times the iron of one fresh banana.

Top Fruit[4] Sources of Youth Enhancing Nutrients

Fruit	Size	Points
Watermelon	10- by 2-inch	10
Papaya	½ medium	9
Cantaloupe	½ medium	8

---

[4]Does not include uncommon fruits which may not be readily available.

Fruit	Size	Points
Mango	½ medium	7
Orange	1 medium	6
Grapefruit	½ medium	5
Banana	1 medium	4
Honeydew melon	7- by 2-inch slice	3
Strawberries	½ cup	2
Pear	1 medium	1

(Based on evaluations from the United Fruit and Vegetable Association and the Center for Science in the Public Interest.)

YOGURT, ACIDOPHILUS AND OTHER CULTURED DAIRY PRODUCTS

In Hindu mythology, the God of Medicine is pictured rising out of an ocean of milk. It has been said that his first command was "Let it be yogurt." So let it be with you.

Are You Eating the Foods of the Gods Every Day?

There may be no old food that helps you live to a ripe old age that's better than yogurt. A staple of the world's youngest old people, including the Hunzas and the Persians—yogurt was called the foods of the gods long before chocolate. According to a Persian tale, an angel taught Abraham how to make it. Some historians even date yogurt back to Neolithic times. Yogurt began, they say, when milk was left to curdle in clay pots.

A Better-than-Milk Source of Age-Proofing Calcium

Yogurt's proof that a super food doesn't have to be elusive or expensive. Yogurt is a food that one-ups that #1 food milk because it not only contains time-fighting calcium and magnesium and B complex, it's a fermented food as well.[5] The calcium it contains is one reason—ounce for ounce it has 10 times more than milk, meat, fish or poultry, and it's in a form that's more readily absorbed. Two low-calorie cups a day is all it takes to satisfy your calcium requirement (800 mg.), says Khem Shahani, Ph.D., professor of Food Science and Technology at the University of Nebraska-Lincoln.

And calcium's critical if you want to put a little more time on your side after 30 or 40. You need that 800 milligrams as a minimum (make that 1200 mg. if you're a woman) a day. The calcium deficiency diseases that go with

---

[5]According to USDA studies, yogurt surpasses low-fat milk in protein, calcium, phosphorus, potassium, zinc, folacin and B-12.

getting older include heart disease, periodontal disease, high blood pressure, cancer and indigestion—and osteoporosis, a disease that leaves bones brittle and vulnerable, peaks during menopause.

Women: Prevent Premature Aging with Breakfast!

According to a 1984 nutrient study by the National Institute on Aging, men, and especially women, tend to consume fewer calcium-rich foods as they age. This disrupts the bone renewal process in the body (20 percent of your skeleton must be replaced annually). This is made worse by a decline in exercise because bone renewal is aided by exercise. The more active you are, says the Aerobics Association of America, the tougher and more calcium-dense your bones become. A yogurt breakfast sundae plus a brisk post-breakfast walk *could* save you from a fractured spine or a dowager's hump or the rocking chair. But that's not all.

Lower Your Cholesterol Level with Yogurt

Besides the calcium it *does* contain, there's the life-shortening fat, cholesterol and calories yogurt *doesn't* contain. According to Dr. Marvin L. Speck, food scientist at North Carolina State University, studies also suggest that yogurt's benefits to longevity may result from what researchers call the "milk factor" which lowers blood cholesterol levels in a way not completely understood. Whatever it is, yogurt has more of it than milk, and this effect may explain the low cholesterol levels and absence of heart diseases among the Masai of East Africa, who live on a cholesterol-rich diet that includes lots of fermented whole milk (yogurt), says Speck.

Yogurt Helps Prevent Candida Infections

Yogurt is a must if you must take antibiotics such as penicillin or tetracycline which tend to kill off the beneficial bacteria that keep your intestinal tract healthy. It also prevents antibiotic-induced diarrhea by recolonizing the gut with beneficial bacteria. Yogurt slows the growth of the virus-causing cold sores (herpes simplex) and vaginal yeast diseases such as candida in older women.

The active bacteria in yogurt also helps start up your digestion by speeding up the breakdown of protein, fat and carbohydrate. And if you have a cry-baby stomach, yogurt's a better way to baby it than milk. It's digested twice as fast as milk, and even if you're milk or lactose-intolerant, chances are you'll tolerate yogurt.

Yogurt—A Rare Source of the Essential Vitamin K

Yogurt's also a good source of that wallflower nutrient vitamin K which a young body produces plenty of but an older one may not. According to researchers at Harvard University, vitamin K helps reduce the loss of calcium from bones that contribute to osteoporosis.

Cancer-free old age may be a benefit of becoming a culture-mover, too. According to researchers Barry Goldin, Ph.D. and Sherwood L. Gorbach, M.D., of the Tufts-New England Medical Center in Boston, high intake of beef and fat has been strongly associated with the risk of developing bowel and colon cancers. When laboratory rats were transferred from a grain to a meat diet, levels of the three enzymes—involved in the formation of these cancer-causing substances in the intestinal tract—rose sharply. "When supplemental lactobacillus acidophilus was added to meat diets, the levels of all three enzymes fell," say the researchers. Two of the enzymes, in fact, fell back to the levels found in animals on a vegetarian diet.

Yogurt Can Help You Unwind During the Day, Sleep Better at Night

Yogurt and cultured milk products are stress-beater foods—providing nerve-soothing B complex and tryptophan, the Valium-alternative amino acid.

Tips for buying yogurt

Here are a few more yogurt facts:

• An 8-ounce serving of non-fat yogurt supplies 130 to 150 calories, but because those calories are in solid form they are more filling than the 150 calories in a glass of whole milk.

• Fruit-flavored yogurts contain sugar and have almost as many calories (260) as a small hamburger on a bun (300).

• Full-fat yogurts contain saturated fats—4 to 11 grams a cup. Lowfat types average 5 grams and nonfat has little or none.

• Yogurt's no great shakes for iron, vitamin A or C or for fiber, but it's richer in B vitamins—especially the anti-fatigue nutrients folic acid and B-12—than milk. If you add fresh fruit and wheat germ you make a cup a meal, says the American Nutritional Consultants Association. And a cupful provides your RDA in protein (20 to 30 percent), calcium (35 to 40 percent), riboflavin (B-2) (20 to 30 percent), vitamin B-12 (15 to 20 percent), phosphorus (25 to 35 percent).

Take a look. Serving size: one 8-ounce cup (227 grams):

	Plain Yogurt (Lower Nonfat)	Flavored Yogurt (coffee, lemon, vanilla)	Fruit Yogurt (strawberry cherry, honey, etc.)
Calories	130–150	200	260
Protein	12 g.	12g.	10 g.

	Plain Yogurt	Flavored Yogurt	Fruit Yogurt
Carbohydrate	17 g.	32 g.	49 g.
Cholesterol			
(mg. per serving)	15 mg.	10–15 mg.	15–20 mg.
(mg. per 100 gm)	5 mg.	5 mg.	5–19 mg.

How Yogurt Is Made

And here's how this "wholly cow" stuff is made: In a yogurt factory, milk is warmed to about 140°F. Any combination of cream, skim or partially skim milk and dry milk solids may be added before the mixture is homogenized and pasteurized. After the milk has cooled to about 115°, it is inoculated with a starter (usually equal amounts of *Lactobacilli* and *Streptococcus* bacteria). The temperature is held for three to six hours to let the culture grow and ferment, then the yogurt is refrigerated to retard fermentation.

There are two basic types of yogurt: *set* and *stirred* (or pudding-style). In *set yogurt*, fermentation occurs right in the retail container. The warm, inoculated mixture is poured in, allowed to ferment, and then cooled. If the product is a flavored sundae-style yogurt, fruit purée or syrup is poured in first.

Stirred yogurts, which includes Swiss and French styles, are fermented in large vats, where they partially coagulate. The yogurt is then stirred back to a fluid, along with any flavoring, to fill the retain containers. In Swiss-style flavored products, a solidifying agent such as gelatin is used. French-style yogurts don't use gelatin, and so are somewhat runnier.

Should you buy your cup of culture for the day or make it? Count on doing both. Supermarket yogurts don't have it all if you're after all the age-proofing nutrients of fermented milk. According to various studies, the more friendly bacteria *L. acidophilus* a yogurt contains (read the label), the better its potential in preventing colitis, constipation, migraine and fatigue, mouth sore and ulcerations and radiation injury—even a beauty aid producing a smoother skin if you use it externally, too. Read labels.

Three foods similar to yogurt are kefir, acidophilus and cultured buttermilk. Kefir is a kind of "sparkling buttermilk" containing yeast cells, which give milk a natural carbonation and produce higher concentrations of B vitamins. Acidophilus milk is a non-fermented dairy drink for the lactose-intolerant. All three supply most of yogurt's benefits.[6]

---

[6]To get more yogurt power into your diet, get it powdered. Yogurt, buttermilk, kefir and acidophilus are all available in dry form (see *Sources*).

Yogurt Alternatives

Even if you are allergic to milk itself rather than just the lactose it contains, there's a "wholly cow-I-can't-believe-this-isn't yogurt" alternative for cow's milk. Yogurt can be made from soybeans or from the milk of non-dairy animals including sheep, goats, yaks and camels or water buffalo, even nuts and seeds. Any good manual on yogurt-making will tell you how.

Why bother to do your own yourself when yogurt-makers are happy to make this longevity food for you? According to the trade journal, *Whole Foods*: "After seven days, the healthful bacteria in yogurt begins to decline; yogurt has a shelf life of 30 days before it begins to mold but commercial yogurt is shipped all over the country at variances of temperature controls with thickeners added. It's doubtful that you're getting what you think you're getting. Additives which may be in commercial yogurt can be avoided and homemade yogurt costs about 10 cents a cup." Here are two simple formulas that don't call for gadgetries.[7]

Easy yogurt #1

A thermos bottle serves as a good yogurt-maker because it maintains a temperature between 90 and 105°F.

• Heat 1 quart of lowfat milk to lukewarm. Stir in 1 tablespoon of fresh, plain storebought yogurt using a whisk or the electric blender.
• Pour cultured milk into a wide-mouthed 1-quart (or larger) thermos. Let set 4 to 6 hours. When thickened, refrigerate in or out of thermos.

Easy yogurt #2

Combine in electric blender:

1 pint half-and-half or fresh cream

2 or 3 tablespoons of cultured buttermilk

• Pour into an earthenware bowl or covered casserole dish. Let set for 6 to 8 hours on top of a warm radiator or in a low oven. When thick, refrigerate.

And once you prepare it, you can make it twice as nutritious by adding any of the following:

• Two tablespoons of chopped dried apricots or ½ cup cubed cantaloupe or peach (all you need to meet your daily A requirements).
• One-half cup of orange/grapefruit/tangerine sections, strawberries or papaya chunks (to double your vitamin C intake).

---

[7]But a gadget like an electric yogurt-maker costs less than $15 and it cultures milk while you sleep. Or get a *Sunpot*, a non-electric cultured food maker that whips up creme fraiche, sour cream, cottage cheese and buttermilk as well (see *Sources*).

• Stir in 1 tablespoon each raisins (chopped dates or prunes) and chopped nuts (to satisfy your daily iron requirements).

When you buy it, here are a few tips:

• Avoid flavored and fruit yogurts. One-half cup of fresh fruit which you can add yourself, only has 50 sugar-free calories a serving. Sugar interferes with the action of yogurt's bacteria.

• Check sodium content. It can run as low as 150 mg or as high as 280 mg.

• Buy only yogurt containing live active bacteria strain. Most such as Dannon do. Some store brands do not.

• Avoid brands with additives which aren't necessary if the original ingredients are first-rate. And yogurts with commercial carageen, a stabilizer, are best avoided during pregnancy and infectious diseases, warns the Consumers Union of Mt. Vernon.

• Check the date on the carton. Refrigerated yogurt will keep seven days, but after seven days its benefits run out.

• The best time and best way to get the most calcium from yogurt is to take it at bedtime with your daily calcium supplement. This prevents calcium which is stored during the day from being lost while you sleep.

Top sources of cultured milks

• Yogurt tablets, powder and capsules
• Fresh yogurt
• Yogurt chips and nuggets (snacks)
• Buttermilk products
• Yogurt drinks
• Kefir liquid
• Kefir milk
• Acidophilus milk
• Acidophilus tablets
• Acidophilus powder
• Kefir-culture powder
• Frozen yogurt
• Powdered buttermilk

SEAWEEDS AND SEA VEGETABLES

Keep your hopes up if you want to stay healthy and have an occasional sea vegetable cocktail. Feeling hopeful heightens your ability to fight disease while depression lowers it, say researchers Drs. Harold and Donna

Udelman at Camelback Hospital, Phoenix. So does the seafood that isn't fish.

Revitalize Your Adrenal Glands with Salt Substitutes

Research by rheumatoid arthritis researchers found lower T-cell production—critical to the immune system—in the depressed patients than in the just as sick but content patients. "Emotions affect the adrenal glands, which secrete cortisol—a hormone that suppresses the body's immune system," says Dr. Udelman.

And what does a sea vegetable cocktail do for longevity? Provides plenty of the brain-perk amino acid phenylalanine—a natural anti-depressant also found in soybeans, chocolate and the sugar substitute aspartame. Sea vegetables are nature's low-sodium (12 percent) alternative to high-sodium (40 percent) salt and much more.

Dr. Bernard Jensen's Health Valley Farm in Arizona serves a rejuvenation sea vegetable salad for lunch, the Pritikin Longevity Center in California recommends sea vegetables for their heart-healthy fiber, and middle-aged marathoners such as Amby Burfoot says his vegetarian diet heavy-on-the-kelp-hold-the-cutlets, is what keeps him in the running.

A Weed with 100 Times the Blood-Building Iron of Spinach

All algaes (seaweeds) are high in calcium, the so-called "milk mineral" that keeps bones younger longer and normalizes blood pressure. If you were an Eskimo athlete running in the Arctic, for example, your diet would contain five times the calcium found in the average American diet. Just 1 ounce of kelp from Eskimo waters provides 273 mg. of calcium, over 25 percent of the Recommended Daily Allowance for this mineral that keeps the heart healthy. Seaweed also supplies energizing iodine and age-proofing vitamins A and B complex (including B-12) plus blood-building iron (100 times more than spinach), anti-cancer beta-carotene, antioxidants such as selenium and trace minerals that boost immune system health—all in easily digestible form, along with sodium alginate, a fiber similar to the pectin in fruit that lowers cholesterol, prevents constipation and helps bind and eliminate toxins such as radioactive strontium 90 from the intestinal tract.

Reduce Your Risk of Post-40 Diabetes, End Constipation and Hypoglycemia

There's more. These good-deed weeds supply the trace mineral chromium essential for keeping blood sugar levels normal, which in turn reduces the risk of age-related ills such as diabetes. There's zinc as well for sexual health and more copper and silicon nutrients (crucial to skin elasticity), and manganese (it helps fight munchies) than anything you're likely to have eaten all week.

Are You Using the World's Richest Source of B-12?

Spirulina, for example, is a salt-and-pepper-tasting microalga (sold in powdered form even at drugstores) which may be the richest source of B-12 known in the plant world. It even surpasses comfrey. Spirulina is 65 percent complete protein—providing 18 of the 22 amino acids. Two tablespoons gives you 6000 I.U. of stay-young, cancer-blocking vitamin A, more B-12 than fried liver and three times the blood-building iron than a diet portion of sirloin steak, with a tenth of the calories. You even get a whopping 1,315 mg. of calcium (more than you get from cottage cheese) and 1,915 mg. of magnesium (more than you get from a magnesium-staple like cashews).

How to Get a "Sugar" Boost with Sea Vegetables

Spirulina builds rather than destroys post-30 periodontal health because it contains two sea vegetable sugars called *rhamnose* and *glycogen* which promote energy without high calories.

Or consider kelp. It thrives in waters that contain up to 200,000,000 tons of dissolved age-proofing minerals per cubic mile. The amount of iodine in kelp exceeds that in land plants like spinach by more than 200 percent; an important point if you've eliminated salt (a source of iodine) and you're eating very little iodine-rich fish. You need iodine for production of intestinal juices to reduce cholesterol and help your body flush out toxic materials. And it's essential for thyroid health, normal estrogen levels, vitamin E utilization and resistance to infection.

Seaweeds Help You Beat the Blahs and the Blues

If you aren't getting enough natural iodine you'll know it. Iodine deficiency causes the blahs, the blues, an inability to metabolize foods efficiently and unexplained weight gains.

Why Doctors Prescribe Sea Vegetables to Prevent and Treat Cancer

Doctors at Johns Hopkins Medical School in Baltimore say an acid in certain types of seaweed resembles the transmitter substance that activates animal nerve cells. They hope to apply it to studies of neuromuscular disorders. And at the Scripps Institute of Oceanography at La Jolla, California, research chemist William Fenical says that seaweed acid also cures stomach cancer in mice and may one day be used to treat human stomach cancers.

In *The Healing Sea*, Dr. George D. Ruggieri and Norman David Rosenberg tell the story of *Tethya crypta*, a Caribbean sponge that led to the development of a widely used anti-cancer drug. While treating a specimen of the sponge with an organic solvent to determine its fat content, Dr. Werner Bergmann and his students at Yale University noticed a strange white substance in the flask. They analyzed the substance and found they had stumbled on unknown members of the class of compounds called nucleotides, the basic building blocks of the nucleic acids RNA and DNA that carry codes governing the growth and reproduction of animal cells. After nine years of research and testing, a compound now extensively used in the treatment of leukemia emerged. Another version of the compound has been found to attack the herpes encephalitus virus.

In addition, seaweed extracts administered after surgery or X-ray treatment to patients with bone cancer have been shown to reduce nausea and fatigue and improve appetites. The algae, *Digenea simplex*, a source of kainic acid, is effective against roundworms, tapeworms and whip worms. In homeopathy, seaweed is routinely used to treat headache, obesity, goiter, flatulence, constipation and high blood pressure.

How You Can Use These Good-Deed Weeds Daily

Uses? You won't believe how many ways there are to use these live-longer ocean greens. *Dulse* and *kelp* make a good 12 percent sodium substitute; *agar* produces low-calorie, high-nutrient puddings, and natural jellos and jellies; *wakame* and *kombu* are the stuff of which high-fiber soups and stews are made; *hiziki* is a good wheat-free pasta substitute, while *arame* is the right stuff for cold salads. *Nori*, a seaweed sold in toast and eaten in parchment-like sheets makes a good, quick aquatic potato chip, as well as a no-fat, near-zero in calories bacon substitute.

Any whole seaweed may be added to soups, casseroles or stews after a brief chopping and soaking. And *all* ocean weeds are good cold in salads or hot in casseroles, in stir-fries and in curries. Or moisten and use in place of lettuce in your next meat-free BLT. And if algae doesn't taste all that good to you, you can hold your nose and take it in liquid extract form.

Sea vegetable researchers say there are at least two dozen commercially sold types of sea produce in all. There's bound to be one you can live with. Here are the goods you get from the seven, which most health food stores, some pharmacies and supermarkets carry:

Nutritional Value of Sea Vegetables

Name	Calcium	Iron	Iodine	Potassium
Agar	567	6.3	0.2	-0-
Dulse	296	150	8	8060
Hijiki	1400	30	-0-	-0-
Irish moss	885	8.9	-0-	2844
(*Chondrus crispus*)				
Kelp	1093	100	150	5273
Nori-green	470	23	-0-	-0-
Nori-red	470	23	-0-	-0-

Top Sources of Live-Longer Sea Vegetables

Sea vegetables sold in ready-to-use, dried form

- Hijiki
- Agar
- Irish Moss (carageen)
- Wakame
- Kelp (powdered or kelp tablets)
- Kombu
- Nori-green (dried or flakes)
- Nori-red
- Dulse—whole, dried or flakes
- Sea vegetable pasta
- Seaweed snack crackers
- Sodium alginate—tablets or liquid
- Spirulina
- Liquid seaweed extract for gardening
- Iodine—tablets or liquid
- Herbal diet formulas

SOYBEANS AND SOYFOODS

If you've got what it takes, why let it get away from you? It won't if you add soybeans to your diet.

22 Ways to Use Low-Fat Soyfoods in Place of High-Fat Meat

The soybean, known as "meat without bones" or "the cow of China" in the Orient, is not one, but several foods in one. Practically a kingdom of superfoods, in fact. Soybeans can be boiled like chestnuts, baked like navy beans, deep-fried like Chinese peas, roasted like peanuts, sprouted like lentils, stir-fried like mungbeans, cultured like yogurt and turned into soy yogurt or tofu; even fermented like cheese and turned into that other all-purpose, low-calorie veal-chicken-and-camembert-cheese substitute, tempeh. Or it can be aged and transformed into soy sauce, teriyaki sauce or aged even more and transformed into the high-protein, all-purpose gravy-maker and seasoning base called *miso*—not to mention non-dairy soybean milk and "ice cream" for the lactose-intolerant (which includes half the plus-50 population) and the milk-allergic (30 percent of the population) as well as low-fat, healthy-heart dieters.

However you use your bean, you get plenty in return. Soybeans are 40 percent protein (twice as high as other beans), and 50 percent protein if you use them in a concentrated form such as soyflour. Just one tablespoon of soyflour added to four tablespoons of corn flour more than doubles the protein content. In either case, there's only 17 percent fat, and it's unsaturated.

Soy protein supplies large amounts of stay-young amino acids comparable to meat, eggs and dairy foods. It is one of the few "good food" sources of the natural appetite-suppressing, mood-elevation, pain-killing amino acid *D-phenylalanine*, and the *only* phenylalanine food besides sea vegetables that's so low in calories. Critics say the amino acid protein balance of soybeans isn't perfect, but even if it isn't, it comes awfully close. Especially when you eat your time-fighting beans with some life-extension puffed wheat, oats or corn.

Increase Your Pep with Soy Foods

With only 2 percent starch, soybeans are richer in potassium—an essential mineral that gives you more live longer pep than any common food with the exception of nutritional yeast. There are 5,000 members of the pulse-legume (beans to you) family, but not a one can touch the soybean for protein. As a non-dairy beverage, enjoyed by milk allergy sufferers and dairy-product-abstaining vegetarians, for example, soy milk supplies 15 times as much iron, 50 percent less fat and only ⅒ of the hazardous agricultural chemical residue found in conventional cow's milk.

What the Japanese Medical Association Says About Soy Milk and Your Heart

The world's most celebrated cholesterol-free "vegetable milk," says the Japanese Medical Association, "is a preferred medical treatment for diabetes and hardening of the arteries because it is so rich in nerve-nourishing lecithin and linoleic acid, and so low in sugar and starch." Try a soy milk smoothie instead of a potent medicine next time you have a post-30's complaint such as diarrhea or constipation. It remedies both.

A soybean a day may even keep gallstones away. According to Dr. David Kritchevsky, associate director of the Wistar Institute who recently conducted animal studies, soy protein cut the level of cholesterol in bile. The less cholesterol, the less likely it is to form into stones.

Soybeans also fight off osteoporosis and arteriosclerosis. Researchers at California's Loma Linda University, studying middle-aged men, indicate that those who eat meat daily are three times as likely to die of a heart attack as their soybean-loving vegetarian contemporaries.

You Get All Six Artery-Cleaning Factors in Soy Foods

In matters of the heart, soya is legume #1. Soybeans are a rich source of three of the six artery-cleaning factors—pectin (a fiber), chromium (a trace nutrient), vitamin C, fish oil, fiber, calcium (mineral)—essential for a healthy older heart. (The only other natural foods that furnish a healthy heart are oranges, strawberries, broccoli and unpeeled potatoes.)

Need a pleasure pick-me-up? Soybeans create a feel-good effect comparable to fructose. (Fructose gets a 20, soybeans a 15.) A tablespoon of soy oil remedies dieter's inertia, too. Laboratory tests have shown that cold-pressed soy oil fed to young rats boosted their energy significantly, and the same results have been observed in two-legged, over-50 athletes suffering from fatigue due to lactic acid buildup in muscle tissue. As a bonus, soy oil has half the fat of hamburgers or eggs.

Tips for Tofu and Tempeh Users

Probably tofu is the tastiest way to use soy. Seven ounces of tofu supplies more than 75 percent of your RDA for age-proof protein (which is either 40 grams or 30 grams depending on whether you agree with the U.S. government or the United Nations guidelines), along with crucial longevity nutrients that meat lacks—vitamin C, fiber and that osteoporosis-blocking mineral, calcium. (One large egg has 27 mg. calcium, one 2 × 2 × 1 inch square of tofu has 131 mg.)

Better tofu is made with calcium salts which increases calcium without adding phosphorus—and when it is prepared this way, it becomes a good source of calcium, low in phosphorus and quite different from the standard American proteins which tend to be high-phosphorus and low-calcium (meat, poultry, fish and processed cheeses).

When you tire of tofu, there's always tempeh. This unique, ready-to-eat soyfood is fermented like vinegar, low in saturated fats, cholesterol and sodium, low in calories and tastes good. In fact, it tastes a lot like chicken or veal, depending on how you fix it, and its protein is comparable to or better than that of poultry and meat dishes.

Tempeh is also the richest known non-animal source of B-12, especially if your digestion is not what it was at 20. More digestible than milk or even fish, it contains enzymes produced during fermenting that break down the bean's rich proteins and oils and tenderize the bean pulp, improving the over-all nutritional value of the bean in the process. Better yet, this vegetarian non-meat treat has only 157 calories per 3½-ounce serving—and, like tofu, it's a multi-purpose fast food. It's even 300 percent cheaper than meat and fish.

Miso, the Gravy-Maker and Tea Substitute That Helps Prevent Hypertension and Cancer

Don't like soybeans as a main dish? Use them as a side dish, and live longer. Miso, a soy paste made by fermenting soybeans with (or without) a whole grain such as barley, and then adding salt and water, has hundreds of uses. Miso-cup, a drink that replaces coffee and soup as a pick-me-up in many Oriental households, is only 12 percent sodium and provides 4 grams of complete protein a serving, and just a fraction of the calories in chicken broth. Miso is said to readjust the alkaline-acid balance in the body, a step that by itself helps fend off lots of age-related diseases. It also supplies important lactic-acid bacteria needed in the small intestine to assure digestion and assimilation of the nutrients in foods. And according to S. Akizuki, M.D. of St. Francis Hospital in Nagasaki, Japan. ". . . Miso belongs to the highest medicine."

According to nutritionist Dr. K. Morishita, miso contains anti-hypertension and anti-arteriosclerosis factors plus zybicolin, which combines with radioactive substances in the body eliminating them through the feces, proving even better that miso is a useful food which can prevent radiation disease.

If you don't like miso—as coffee or tea—use it as a live-longer, low-sodium sauce base and gravy-starter to add calcium, phosphorus, iron, potassium, magnesium and selenium to your menu. It even contains a large amount of natural glucose for quick candy-bar-like energy.

Soybean products have long served as man's best known source of lecithin, too, a nerve, brain and diet food. Lecithin is found in all the body's living cells and it promotes digestion of fats, prevents fat buildup on artery walls and helps lower the concentration of cholesterol and other fats in the bloodstream. Besides that, it's a sex-after-60 essential because it helps manufacture the hormone in sperm.

Boost Your Brain Power with Ice Cream "Sprinkles"

Lecithin supplements are obtained commercially from soybeans. Lecithin is sold in liquid, powder and granulated form. (About one-third of the liquid form is soybean oil and the rest is lecithin. Because of the oil content, this is a higher-in-calories form of lecithin.) A second way to get your daily life-extension dose of lecithin is from supplements. One tablespoon of granules or five high-potency capsules usually supplies 1,200 milligrams of lecithin. Or use lecithin granules, which add a ground-nut-like flavor to ice cream, cereal, salads, and soups, or mix into juices, sauces, baking batters, soups, salad dressings, and juices.

If you decide to have a plate of tofu rather than beef or cheese, here are a few of the dietary essentials you stand to lose or gain:

Nutrients	Firm Tofu	Beef	Cheese
Calories	112.50	161.0	315.00
Protein (g.)	12.00	26.6	19.80
Saturated fat (g.)	0.90	2.5	14.10
Unsaturated fat (g.)	5.10	2.7	11.40
Cholesterol	0.00	80.0	78.00
Calcium (mg.)	36.00	11.0	594.00
Iron (mg.)	2.70	3.1	0.00

Richest sources of soybeans

- Dried soybeans
- Canned soybeans
- Tofu (soybean curd)
- Tempeh (fermented meat substitute)[8]
- Cracked and flaked dried soybeans (for casseroles)
- Soybean sprouts
- Miso (soybean paste)
- Soy sauce (regular and low-sodium)
- Soy lecithin (granules and powder)
- Liquid lecithin (a vegetable oil)[8]
- Soy milk drinks[8]
- Soy milk powder
- Canned soy milk
- Soybean flour
- Soy grits
- Soy pasta (spaghetti, macaroni, etc.)
- Soy granules
- Soy cereal flakes
- Texturized soy protein[8] (for making "mock meats")
- Miso-cup (a tea/coffee/soup substitute)[8]
- Soy (non-dairy) ice cream, yogurt and frozen desserts
- Prepared soy main dishes, frozen and canned,[8] such as tofu lasagna, etc.

---

[8]At health food stores and large supermarkets.

• Processed supermarket foods containing lecithin and soy byproducts

WHOLE GRAIN BREADS AND CEREALS

Methuselah lived 900 years. Whole grains were probably half the
reason. One out of every 300 Abkhuzians in the USSR is over 100, and the
one food they eat daily is a cornmeal mush bread called Abrusta.

The Live-Longer Factor in Whole Grains

Grains can do a lot for *your* young-old-timer status, too. They are a
good source of energizing carbohydrate, vitamin B complex and a top
source of all the time-fighting antioxidants except ascorbic acid (vitamin
C)—but most of all, they contain live-longer fiber. Snacking on wheat
rather than a sweet pays off in the prevention of many mid-life ills. According to Dr. Denis Burkitt of the Medical Research Council in England, it's
wheat that prevents and sugar that contributes to the increased risk of
diabetes, the blindness which often results from it, obesity, digestive disorders such as diverticulosis, appendicitis, hemorrhoids, varicose veins and
hiatus hernia, even rectal tumors and heart disease. All these diseases are
in great part due to the fact that our diets are too low in whole grains and
too high in sugar.

Four Types of Fiber for Super-Health

Whole grains (breads, cereals and sprouts are a few sources) actually
supply four out of the six major types of do-good fiber: lignin, gums,
cellulose and hemicellulose. The other two are pectin, the fiber that turns
fruit juices into jelly—found almost exclusively in vegetables and fruits
such as apples and grapes—and beta-glucan found in beans. It is slightly
less laxative.

The rough stuff in grain we call fiber is health stuff because it blocks
carcinogens in the intestinal tract, prevents constipation, controls appetite
and normalizes weight. It also protects against gallstone formation, bile
acid-cholesterol buildup, says authority Dr. Peter Van Soest, Cornell University's nutritionist and fiber researcher. What's good for your middle-
aged digestion is even good for your middle-aged complexion. "Fiber
interacts with poisonous substances in the feces to prevent their absorption
into the circulation," says Burkitt. "When they are efficiently eliminated
instead of being absorbed, clear skin, shiny hair and a sweeter breath
result." (If you're a 150-pound male you need 37 grams of fiber a day to get
such believe-it-or-not benefits—have a cup of cold bran cereal and toast in
the morning and two cups of hot popcorn at night.)

How Whole-Grain Fiber Helps Control Cholesterol and Prevent Cancer

Here's how the nutritional defense mechanisms of fiber work. Fiber improves the consistency and bulk of the stool (feces) and the time it takes to go through the intestines. It moves the stool more quickly through the bowels, so bowel tissues, as a result, have a reduced exposure to toxins and the cancer-causing substances which, says Burkitt, are always being produced in the intestines as food is broken down and excreted.

Fiber helps reduce the amount of cholesterol you absorb from food and alters the amount of cholesterol which is manufactured by your liver, thus reducing your risk of heart disease. Grains can be just as good, as long as the bran and germ are there. Your morning mush, for example, can be oatmeal, and again, fiber gets the credit.

Why Doctors Recommend a Bowl of Cereal to Start Your Day

"One-half cup of dry oat bran worked into an otherwise typical American diet can lower LDL cholesterol levels (bad cholesterol) by as much as 25 percent within as few as 10 days," says Dr. James Anderson, professor of medicine and nutrition at the University of Kentucky. The water-soluble fiber that makes oatmeal gummy is beta glucan. This special fiber is also present in legumes such as pinto, navy and soybeans.

Surprising Sources of Bran if You Can't Have Wheat

Oat bran also regulates blood sugar levels in diabetics. Or try millet, a crunchy rice/corn substitute (more digestible than either and lower in calories) that's rich in iron, magnesium, potassium and protein that makes good mush and a better-than-cornbread muffin. Or, farther afield—amaranth, an exceptionally rich source of calcium, iron and vitamin C, potassium, vitamin A, riboflavin, niacin and an above-average source of protein. (Amaranth was once the staple food of the Mayan and Aztec Indians and can be traced back to 6000 B.C. or even earlier.) Cultivated in the Far East, Africa, Mexico and some tropical countries as well as the U.S., it's available in health food stores and by mail as a graham cracker, ready-to-eat cereal, a flour and a seed for sprouting.

Are You Eating a High-Energy Breakfast?

All whole grains are good energizers because the B-1 they contain acts as a co-enzyme in dozens of the body's enzyme systems to reduce the post-exercise lactic acid buildup in body tissues which produces fatigue. Whole grains also supply a substance called prostaglandins which help keep hormone levels normal. Grains provide energy in the form of carbohydrate which is more quickly available to the body than the energy in eggs (in the form of protein), for example. Here are the "energy effects" of a grain versus an egg breakfast:

Breakfast #1	Calories	Protein	Energy Effects
1 cup oat-meal with ½ cup skim milk	178	9 g.	Filling and good for fiber but not enough fat to hold your energy for more than 3 hours. Add butter to the cereal or have toast and increase the milk. Fruit will supply extra calories and energy.

Breakfast #2	Calories	Protein	Energy Effects
2 large eggs sunny-side up	240	13 g.	Enough protein and fat to hold you for 4 hours. For quicker, more accessible energy and extra calories, add toast and juice.

How Whole Grains Reduce Stress and Tone Your Nervous System

Another reason to butter up with whole grains for better body health after 30 is stress reduction. According to the world's foremost trace mineral authority, Henry A. Schroeder, physical work, surgical intervention, injury, burns and infections all cause stress. Double your pantothenic acid (B-5) requirement. "A diet with a 25 percent deficiency in pantothenate can damage the central nervous system in only six months," says Dr. Klaus Pietrzik of the Federation of American Societies for Experimental Biology. Grains are a first-choice source of B-5 as well as the rest of the longevity complex, and provide minerals you're bound to be short on—if you're no longer shy of 40. A 3-ounce slice of pumpernickel bread gives you as much calcium and magnesium as a quarter cup of dry-curd cottage cheese. So does a half cup of bulgur wheat plus more iron, and fewer calories than you think. A slice of whole grain bread averages 60 to 70 calories; a half cup of cooked cracked wheat, buckwheat or wild rice has only 60 to 80 calories, less than the 115 in white rice. And because there's more fiber and protein, they satisfy the appetite longer.

As for bran? There are new better-than-wheat-bran and wheat germ possibilities on the shelf, too. Try rice bran, oat bran, soy bran (soy middlings) or corn germ[9]—a crunchier alternative with 10 times the zinc, three times the magnesium and eight times the niacin of wheat germ and bran. Or barley fiber powder,[9] with twice the fiber of wheat germ and more copper, iron, niacin and magnesium than wheat bran or pea bran,[10] has three times the fiber of wheat and is an excellent supply of iron, zinc and magnesium. All brans make good cooked cereals, great breads or tasty sprinkles for salads, soups and sundaes.

10 Top Breads for Health After 30

Here are a few of the live-longer nutrients in your daily bread:

Bread (per 2 oz.)	Dietary fiber (g.)	Magnesium	Zinc	Vitamin B-6	Folacin
Whole wheat	3.2	11	8	3	8
Pumpernickel	3	7	5	3	3
Whole wheat pita	2.7	11	6	8	9
Rye	2.4	5	4	3	6
Cracked wheat	2.2	7	5	2	4
Mixed grain	2.1	8	5	3	9
Oatmeal	1.2	5	4	3	3
French	1.1	3	3	1	4
Italian	0.6	3	3	1	4
Corn tortilla	1.9	9	9	4	2

Tips

1. To improve the fiber levels in bread, toast it, say Cornell University scientists.

2. Be a smart sandwich bread shopper. Standard pumpernickel loaves contain 38 percent rye meal, 38 percent dark rye flour and 24 percent enriched white flour. Rye bread is 60 to 80 percent white flour and 20 to 40 percent medium rye flour. Pumpernickel's coarse rye meal is less refined than flour and its higher total rye content makes it the more nutritious alternative.

3. Corn tortillas are reasonably good as bread substitutes, but they have less iron because they aren't "enriched." Two ounces provide only 4

---

[9]See *Sources.*
[10]See *Sources.*

percent of the U.S. Recommended Daily Allowance for the mineral, rather than the 7 to 10 percent in most breads.

4. The eight best supermarket cereals you can buy (based on fat, salt, sugar and nutrients levels): Shredded Wheat (Quaker, Nabisco); Quick or Old-Fashioned Oats (Quaker, Ralston); Instant or Regular Ralston (Ralston); Cream of Wheat, Regular or Instant (Nabisco); Grape-Nuts Flakes or Regular (Post); Nutri-Grain (Kellogg's); Puffed Rice or Wheat (Quaker); Regular Instant Oats (Quaker). The eight worst: Corn Flakes (Kellogg's, Post, Ralston); Instant Oats with Cinnamon Spices (Quaker); Raisin Bran (Ralston); Alpha-Bits (Post); Froot Loops or Frosted Flakes (Kellogg's); Lucky Charms (General Mills); Cookie Crisp (Ralston); Cap'n Crunch (Quaker).

Top sources of whole grains

• Whole grains (to cook for hot cereals and cold salads): bulgur wheat, barley (non-pearled), buckwheat groats, couscou, wild rice, brown rice, converted white rice, triticale, millet, etc.

• Ready-to-eat supermarket cereals such as shredded wheat, puffed rice, bran flakes, etc.

• Whole-grain flour, ready-to-eat health food store cereals such as puffed corn and puffed rice, unsweetened granola, soy flakes, etc.

• Hot cereals such as oatmeal, cream of rye, seven-grain cereal, corn meal, oat bran, etc.

• Whole grains for sprouting: wheat, rye, rice, etc.

• Whole-grain breads, crackers and snack chips

• Bran and germ supplements.

EVERYDAY FOODS THAT HELP YOU LOOK 10 TO 12 YEARS YOUNGER

Fast foods to help slow down the fast-forward effect at your waistline, hairline, indeed your lifeline? Try sauerkraut or sardines. According to the late biochemist and rejuvenation expert Dr. Benjamin Frank,[11] a diet based on fermented foods (such as kraut) and nucleic acid foods (such as sardines) can take as much as six years off your life if you're 40, and "an elderly person can expect to look and feel 10 to 12 years younger."

---

[11]See the Stay Young Diet based on Dr. Frank's favorite foods under *Menu Plans*, page 73.

How Sauerkraut and Sourdough Prevent Colitis, Ulcers and Hemorrhoids

Fermented foods help keep the supply of "good" bacteria (or intestinal flora) flourishing in your intestines. That's good because, according to gerontologists such as the University of California's Roy L. Walford, it tends to taper off with age. And the more you've got the better your defense against the so-called auto-intoxication of the intestines and colon, a condition that can lead to such stomach disorders as chronic constipation, colitis, ulcers and hemorrhoids.

Are You Eating What the World's Healthiest Old People Eat?

Fermented foods of one kind or another are the meat-and-potatoes of the world's youngest, healthiest old-timers. Japan's Okinawans, who have the highest rate of centenarians in the world, feast on a variety of fermented beans including miso, the soybean paste you can use as a gravy master, beverage-base or bread spread. The American Indian has his pemmican; Alaskans eat briny fish, and sourdough; Russians relish pickled eggs and borsht; Indonesians who live longer do it with a soybean steak and cheese substitute called tempeh; while Americans stay young with the cultured dairy food called yogurt (culturing is a form of fermentation).

The Magic of Nucleic Acid Foods

As for nucleic acid foods,[12] to make this long nutrient story short, according to Dr. Frank, the two nucleic acids, RNA and DNA,[13] improve the ability of your body cells to manufacture and distribute energy for cell functions. They also repair cells that degenerate with aging. The body has rich supplies of RNA and DNA at birth, but after 30, they begin a sharp, steady decline.

"The two body organs that suffer the most from nucleic acid deficiency are the brain and the immune system," say researchers at the Weizman Institute of Science in Israel, which is why such foods as brewer's and nutritional yeast, sweetbreads and sardines—the three best food sources of nucleic acids—might be considered aids in preventing Alzheimer's Disease, arthritis, and cancer. There is no medical consensus that feasting on nucleic acid-rich fish and fermented foods will keep you disease-free from mid-life on—but such foods are rich vitality-boosting, low-calorie sources of protein, and B-complex, especially choline. According to

---

[12]*Note*: Many fermented foods are also nucleic acid foods and vice versa. Pickled herring is a case in point. So is borsht.

[13]DNA is the body's master biochemical blueprint for building new cells. RNA is the "messenger" chemical that carries out the DNA's work in this life process among the cells. RNA forms enzymes the body needs but if aging causes DNA with poorly formed RNA, enzyme formation and metabolism suffers.

1985 reports by Duke University researchers, one of the three causes of senility is a deficiency of choline in brain tissue.

Beat the Flu and the Common Cold with Brewer's Yeast

Dr. Frank notes that more nucleic acids in your diet should raise your immunity to respiratory problems including colds and the flu. For best results, try combining a nucleic acid supplement (30 mg. is good) and one or more servings of foods from the nucleic acid/fermented food groups in your diet. To cover your fermented food bets at the same time, have yeast sprinkled on sardines, beets or sourdough toast. Even if you don't *get* younger, you'll *feel* more youthful zest.

What the USDA Says About the Special Benefits of Brewer's Yeast

As for nutritional and brewer's yeast, life-extension UCLA gerontologist Roy L. Walford, M.D., wouldn't start his day without it. One reason? Yeast is our #1 source of chromium—a trace mineral that protects you from heart attacks by normalizing blood cholesterol levels and from diabetes by improving glucose tolerance, says the Human Nutrition Center of the USDA.

The #1 Way to Get More Chromium for Staying Young

A single serving of most meats, fish, poultry, dairy products, vegetables, fresh fruit, breads, cereals and nuts provides only about 1 to 5 micrograms of chromium, not much considering that the National Academy of Sciences recommends that an adult consume 50 to 200 micrograms per day. Here's what several widely available brands of brewer's yeast provide:

Brand	Chromium (mcg.) in 10 g Yeast
Nature Most	60
Nature Ade	60
Lewis Labs	60
Solgar	60
KAL	22
Plus	16
Vita Food	6

Another reason to add yeast to your menu: It's the second best source of the B vitamin Biotin (liver is #1), a help in preventing such common middle-aged complaints as diarrhea, dysentery and skin trouble. Weight specialist H. L. Newbold calls it "the single most potent rejuvenative food I know."

Do You Need a B-Vitamin Brewer's Yeast Boost?

Yeast also gets credit for speedy recovery from constipation, heart troubles, eczema, dry and scaly skin, dandruff, acne, canker sores, impotency, bloodshot eyes, gallstones, even cirrhosis of the liver. Do you need it? Take a look at your tongue. If it's blue or white and lacey around the edges, you're deficient in the B vitamins brewer's yeast is rich in.

Yeast aids the pancreas by supplying B-6 and zinc, two nutrients American soil is poor in and the reason so many middle-aged among us have low or high blood sugar. It helps your body assimilate the natural sugars in fruits, grains, vegetables, honey and other syrup sweeteners.

Yeast: The World's Oldest Super Food

Max Fleischmann made baker's yeast popular in the United States and not only advertised it for baking but promoted it as a food to help maintain health and youth. Although similar dried brewer's yeast is not identical, it has a nutritional content four times richer than baker's yeast. Good brewer's yeast is a beneficial bacteria that is specially grown on a variety of cultures including dairy whey and blackstrap molasses. Sold in all health food stores, supermarkets and pharmacies, it dissolves readily in liquids (grape or grapefruit improve the flavor best) and keeps a year or longer without refrigeration.

How to add brewer's yeast to your daily meals

1. Add small amounts to baked goods, soups, stews and casseroles.
2. Add 1 or 2 teaspoons to fruit or vegetable juices. (Optional: 1 teaspoon calcium gluconate or bone meal supplies calcium which unfortified yeast lacks.) Drink slowly for a quick energy lift.
3. Add to a glass of skim milk with 1 teaspoon of molasses or honey.
4. Stir 2 tablespoons into cottage cheese or yogurt, low-fat puddings or frozen fruit or dairy desserts.
5. Add to blender fruit-and-milk smoothies.
6. Add to breading mixtures for sautéed and batter-fried foods.
7. Turn it into a chip dip (see recipes).
8. Add powdered calcium to brewer's yeast drinks, or take calcium tablets to help digest the large amounts of phosphorus yeast contains.
9. Use yeast between meals unless you are having a protein-free meal so that sufficient gastric juices are available for digestion.

If you experience bloating or gas, add a hydrochloric acid tablet (HCl) to aid digestion. Bloating will stop as your gastro-intestinal health improves. Gas is a tipoff that you're B-vitamin deficient.

If you notice a tingling or flushing of the skin, that's due to a dilation in the blood vessels caused by the B-vitamin niacin in the brewer's yeast which stimulates the circulation. This is annoying, but a healthy sign.

If you hate the taste of brewer's yeast, buy clear gelatin capsules at the pharmacy or health food store and fill them by hand with powdered yeast.

Top Sources of Nucleic Acids and Fermented Foods

- Brewer's yeast, powder, flakes, or tablets, has twice the nucleic acid content of sardines, the #2 source
- Sardines
- Sweetbreads and other organ meats
- anchovies, salmon, shrimp, oyster, crab, clams, lobster
- Bee pollen, raw honey, honeycomb, propolis, royal jelly
- dried beans and lentils
- B-complex tablets
- RNA/DNA supplements
- Sourdough bread
- Vinegar
- Soybean tempeh (fermented soybean and miso, fermented soy paste, soy sauce)
- Tofu and tofu byproducts such as Tofutti frozen desserts
- Cultured buttermilk
- Acidophilus milk, kefir
- Sour cream
- Ripened cheeses such as Brie, Camembert
- Pickled foods (cabbage, cucumbers, beets, eggs, etc.).
- Beef jerky and fish jerky (pemmican)
- Marmite (a seasoning base based on concentrated yeast)
- Kyolic supplements (a specially aged yeast-garlic supplement)

Top Sources of Brewer's Yeast

- Brewer's yeast
- Powders, flakes, granules, buds
- Yeast tablets
- Liquid herbal yeast
- Yeast extract concentrates such as marmite, vegemite (use as sandwich spread, flavored butter, gravy master), and Bakon (smoked powdered yeast)
- Selenium supplements
- Liver and yeast formula supplements

- Lecithin-yeast capsules
- GTF and chromium supplements
- Natural ingredient B vitamins

ROOT VEGETABLES

"Ten or 12 out of every 100,000 Americans will live to be 100, of which at least one-third will be physically active, mentally alert and free of any major disease," says Dr. John S. Thompson at the University of Kentucky. You improve your chances of being among the numbered if you improve your intake of root vegetables.

Recapturing your lost-and-found youth may be more a matter of less meat and more potatoes, to say nothing of more parsnips, carrots, beets— than it is of Geritol or Gervitol.

Six All-Star Vegetables with the Best Artery-Cleansing Effect

According to the National Cancer Institute, root vegetables such as Brussels sprouts and broccoli with less than 50 calories a cup are good sources of the anti-cancer factor called crucifers or indoles, as well as cancer-fighting beta-carotene—something neither meat, fish nor poultry provide. And on a checklist of foods containing the six all-star artery-cleaning factors (pectin, chromium, vitamin C, fish oils, fiber and calcium), root vegetables are tops, says Julian M. Whitaker, director of the National Heart and Diabetes Treatment Center in Huntington Beach, California.

The Nucleic Acid Staying Young Diet That Helps You Look and Feel Better in Two Weeks

Root vegetables—especially celery and beets—also increase your body's reserve of stay-young nucleic acids. And "nucleic-acid-rich diets have been observed to lower blood cholesterol levels . . . their absence in a diet results in premature aging," advised the late rejuvenation expert Dr. Benjamin S. Frank. (See page 73 for the *Nucleic Acid Anti-Aging Diet*.)

Root vegetables are as high (or higher) in live-longer fiber and life-extension minerals than fruits and grains, so a bowl of borsht has a better satisfy-the-appetite-potential than fast-food fruit pies and provides only half the get-fat calories.

What Cornell University Nutritionists Say About the Youth Factor in Potatoes

If you hate cabbage and beets, you can get younger with more potatoes. The potato is a 100-calorie package of 99.9 percent fat-free, low-sodium nutritional perfections. It has seven of the eight essential amino acids, supplies 33 percent of your RDA for time-fighting vitamin C, plus it contains iron, calcium, zinc, potassium and fiber, and over 1,000 live-longer enzymes, says spud-loving[14] Cornell nutrition researcher Nell Mondy.

The only time potatoes *aren't* a hot line to prime-of-life health is when they're poorly prepared or green. Potatoes contain small amounts of a natural nerve toxin called glycoalkaloids, and green, warm or bruised spuds may have two or three times more of this substance than healthy spuds—enough to cause an eater drowsiness, headache, diarrhea, even high blood sugar, says Mondy. So do right by them.

Deep frying takes a back seat to baking or boiling. Baking causes the nutrients concentrated in the skin to "migrate" toward the center (that's good)—while frying not only quadruples the calories (the boiled potato has 90 calories, fries have 400), but also reduces fiber and masks the bitter taste of high levels of poisonous glycoalkaloids. Potatoes can even be eaten raw. Get into the habit of grating a small amount into every soup or salad you serve.

How Horseradish and Carrots Protect Your Heart and Vision

Another root to root for is horseradish (the word means "sea radish"). Prescribed since medieval times, it's high in vitamin C—and fresh or bottled, they are a good source of the blood pressure-stabilizing trace mineral sulphur (also found in garlic).

To use more of the root you raise or buy, make *Horseradish Mayo* and use it as a saucey, salt-free sour cream substitute: Combine 1 cup sour cream (or *50-Plus Creme Fraiche*, page 114) with 3 tablespoons of freshly grated horseradish. Blend well. Use as a dip, spread, sauce or spud topping.

Last but not least—there are carrots. Chief among dieter's foods, a carrot's color is a sign that it's a source of the substance called carotene. There are 6,000 units of vitamin A in one 5½-inch carrot (only liver has more) plus B-1 and B-2, lots of natural sodium, calcium, some protein, iodine and enzymes (in the raw juice). And if you eat or use the tops, you get iron and vitamin C as well as E. Twenty slim sticks have only 30 crunchy calories and twice the fiber of leafy greens or legumes.

Best live-longer root vegetables

- Carrots
- Potatoes
- Parsnips
- Celery
- Beets

---

[14]Spuds and milk alone—supplying most of the nutrients the body needs— were the staple of the 19th century diet in Ireland.

- Horseradish
- Radishes
- Parsley root
- Celery root
- Turnips
- Jicama
- Garlic
- Kohlrabi

GARLICS, ONIONS

Inside every older person there's a younger person trying to get out. More onions, garlic and alliums of all kinds (the allium family includes scallions, stalk and green onions, Bermuda onions, shallots, leeks and more) could help.

The onion figures prominently in most stay young diets. In the Hunzan valley, one of the world's six hot spots for longevity, onions (and garlic) are eaten daily and there is a virtual absence of heart disease and cancer.

Onions to Reduce Inflammations, Allergic Reactions and Block Asthma

According to University of Munich's Dr. Walter Dorsch, drinking onion juice before exposure to irritants often reduces bronchial asthma attacks up to 50 percent. And an onion juice solution rubbed on arms exposed to contact allergens delays and reduces swelling and inflammation nine out of 12 times. (Onion oil inhibits formation of the prostaglandins in the bloodstream which encourages the allergic reactions.) The one responsible ingredient may be the mustard oils, or isothiocyanates. Onions often have a similar anti-inflammatory magic in cases of rheumatoid arthritis.

Besides isothiocyanates, onions fight diabetes, wrinkles and cancer because they contain a second major ingredient called diphenylamine which helps normalize diabetic blood sugar levels. (The onions with the healthiest levels of diphenylamine are beberis.)

Sulphur—the Cancer-Blocking Trace Mineral in Onions and Garlic

A third ingredient is the trace mineral sulphur (also supplied by garlic)—essential for youthful looking hair, skin and nails, and much more. Research indicates, for example, that onions have the ability to ward off cancer in early stages. "Onion and garlic oils actually inhibit the 'initiation stage' (where an interaction occurs with a normal cell). Components in onions block some of the enzymes necessary to convert a cancer-causing carcinogen into a dangerous chemical," they say. Sulphur gets the credit.

In addition, the onion has few calories, is a fair source of fiber (8 grams) and provides vitamins B-1, B-2 and A. If you're not much on onions, buy one you can munch. The Georgia Vidalia, Washington State Walla Walla or Hawaiian Maui are three varieties sweet enough to eat raw like apples (see *Sources*).

Another source of root vegetable anti-cancer and anti-aging sulphur, if you're avoiding the rocking chair, is garlic. Dr. Gerhard Schrauzer, professor of chemistry at the University of California at San Diego, describes garlic as "a simple, non-prescription drug that helps detoxify the body and prevent disease." What kind of disease? The ones most often associated with aging such as high blood pressure and diabetes.

Garlic is as good an earth medicine as you're likely to find. Used as a cure and a culinary for 4,000 years, garlic has been an important healing agent for the Chinese, Hebrews, Egyptians, Greeks, Romans and Hindus. It was found in the tomb of Egyptian King Tutankhamen and was consumed by laborers who built the Great Pyramid. Muhammed used garlic to treat scorpion stings. It is mentioned in clay tablets found in Nineveh (circa 668 to 626 B.C.) and cited by the Hebrews' Talmud for satiating hunger and improving circulation.

The average midlife American eats five times more garlic now than 15 years ago. And that still doesn't make us tops—the Thais, Koreans and Greeks eat the largest amounts of what botanists and gardeners affectionately call "the stinkin' rose" (garlic and roses are related).

Allicin: The-Better-than-Drugs Remedy for High Cholesterol, Hypertension and Headaches

According to researchers in Cologne, Germany, garlic helps clear fat from blood cells. Tests show that diners fed garlic in gelatin capsules had considerably lower cholesterol levels than those of a control group fed butter without garlic. In other tests where garlic was used on patients with abnormally high blood pressure, hypertension was lowered by 45 percent. Further, dizziness, angina pains and headaches also disappeared with garlic therapy.

Fight 15 Infections with Onions and Garlic

Here's why: According to the American Herb Trade Association, garlic supplies at least two natural anti-bodies or germ killers that act against 15 species of harmful bacteria. It stimulates the pituitary gland in the brain to prevent glandular slowdown that results in memory loss and declining gastrointestinal functions, and garlic has allicin—the substance that is believed to be largely responsible for garlic's anti-bacterial and anti-inflammatory effects.

Small a plant though it is, garlic also supplies big-gun biological benefits. Here are a few of the components and factors it contains, one of which you're bound to need:

• *Gurwitch Rays*, the mitogenetic radiation factor that stimulates cell growth and rejuvenates all body functions.

• *An Anti-Hemolytic Factor*, responsible for garlic's effectiveness in treating anemia.

• *Selenium*, the factor believed to be responsible for garlic's clot-formation-prevention potential.

• *Anti-Toxin*, which helps detoxify the digestive tract and fortify the body's defenses against allergies and asthma.

And since it tastes good, has nearly no calories and makes a super substitute for salt, and fights indigestion better than antacids, it couldn't hurt to eat garlic daily. Best results come from large, regular doses. When considering garlic as a supplement, look for high potency—and to benefit from all the nutrients and trace minerals, a cold-processed, enzyme-active garlic is best. Another way to benefit? Use your garlic in juices.

Is garlic too strong for your taste? Eat sprigs of raw parsley or chew fennel or caraway seeds. Cooking also neutralizes the odor. Or switch to a mild-flavored Oriental or elephant garlic (see *Sources*) which have milder flavors.

Both onion and garlic are best used fresh. And use them in as many forms as you can find. It helps to know your leeks from your onions. Leeks look like overgrown scallions (green onions) and are usually cooked, scallions are eaten raw, while shallots are a mild-mannered kind of "carriage trade" onion worth a try if you cook a lot and use a lot of onions. With the exception of dried bulb types, all should be refrigerated.

As an herbal bonus—either allium can be potted. The sprouts that appear make good chive substitutes. The best way to get the most good out of garlic is to take it daily with vitamin E and F (vegetable oils) to increase its potency in your system. In turn, you will benefit by improved absorption of energizing B-1.

Three basic ways to get both good alliums into your diet: Homemade purées, butters and oils (see recipes in *Spreads*).

Top sources of garlic

• Garlic purée (sold in vacuum-packed jars in supermarket fresh produce section, or see recipe, page 105)
• Dried garlic bulbs
• Garlic capsules and tablets (with or without parsley)
• Kyolic capsules (aged garlic fortified with vitamins and nutritional yeast)

- Elephant garlic
- Garlic/parsley tablets
- Garlic flakes
- Garlic powder (*not* garlic salt)

Top sources of onions

- Fresh onions, all bulbs and stalk varieties
- Dried onions in flakes, granules and powder
- Onion powder (*not* onion salt)
- Herb salt substitutes
- Dried-soup vegetable flakes

Your body is engineered for more than three score and 10, says Swedish gerontologist Dr. Alvar Svanburg, and if you get more sprouts into your daily diet, you might just make it, too. Sprouts are a good source of 10 of the top 12 age-proofing nutrients, supply fiber and have fewer calories, short of celery.

Why the National Heart and Diabetes Institute Puts Alfalfa Sprouts on the Menu

Make the sprouts alfalfa, a super food even supermarkets supply, for example, and your lease on life can be longer because your heart will be hardier. What's alfalfa's magic? There's evidence, says the National Heart and Diabetes Institute, that it may be able to raise the ratio of high-density lipoproteins (HDL) to low-density lipoproteins (LDL). This ratio is a measure of the balance between HDL, the factor that helps carry cholesterol out of the system, and LDL, the material that helps keep cholesterol intact. The higher the ratio, the better. "Alfalfa seeds are a key part of our Healthy Heart Diet," says Dr. Julian M. Whitaker, M.D., director of the NHDI in Huntington Beach, California. "We serve alfalfa at every meal."

Sprouts supply vitamins C, E and B in their full complex. These three nutrients are noted for their cholesterol-stabilizing effect and more. Sprouts also give you a daily dose of the blood-clotting factor known as vitamin K which also helps your body maintain its calcium reserves—good news if you hate the usual good sources of vitamin K, such as liver and turnip greens.

Sprouts Give You More Vitamins and Minerals than Other Foods

Sprouting improves the nutrients in any seeds food. Sprouting dried peas, for example, increases their vitamin C content by 800 percent in four days, says America's number-one sprout authority, Jeff Breakey. In lentils and mung beans, vitamin C content triples along with vitamin C. Unsprouted wheat kernels have only 28 grams of the anti-anemia B vitamin, folic acid. Sprouting increases it to 106 grams. What's true for wheat is true for any other seeds you germinate for now-and-later-life food health.

Sprouts May Help Prevent Cancer

Sprouted wheat could help you beat cancer, suggests biologist Chiu-Nan Lai at the M.D. Anderson Hospital and Tumor Institute. "Extracts of sprouts, particularly from wheat, counteract carcinogens . . . Research studies show that chlorophyll accounts for most of the extract's anti-cancer effect . . ."

All sprouts contain some percentage of chlorophyll, the substance that gives plants their green color and the energy to carry on the process of photosynthesis. Chlorophyll is chemically related to hemoglobin in the human blood. (The only difference being that chlorophyll contains magnesium, while the blood contains iron.) Chlorophyll helps build blood, aids digestion, stimulates tissue growth and freshens the breath.

It also can literally save your skin, say dermatologists such as Albert M. Klyna, director of Pennsylvania Aging Skin Clinic. Sprouts provide you with six nutrients that prevent three tell-tale signs of age—dry skin, gray hair and receding gums. Those nutrients are calcium, zinc and vitamins A, D, B and E.

Put Zip in Your Life for Zero Calories

Sprouts even supply a "40-and-feeling-good" substance called aspartic acid[15] that provides a "natural hormonal high," says biochemist Dr. Roger Williams. ". . . One means of determining stamina is to force an animal to swim until exhausted . . . and note the swimming time. It is by this means that it has recently been found that the amino acid aspartic acid is possibly of greater nutritional importance than has been previously suspected. Administering salts of this acid to rats . . . doubles the length of time they can swim before exhaustion. Corroboration of this increase in stamina has been reported in the case of athletes also . . ."

And despite their low-calorie content (40 to 100 calories a cup), sprouts are high energy foods. Like potatoes and pasta, they are rich in fiber and complex carbohydrates, but the natural fruit and vegetable sugars they contain are in the form of simple monosaccharides like that in honey and fruit which enter the bloodstream rapidly and provide a fast lift.

Sprouted foods are easier to digest because they come packaged with their own digestive enzymes. Good news for post-40 stomachs which tend to run low on enzymes and hydrochloric acid. (Your body has billions of

---

[15]Aspartic acid is also found in the pits of almonds, apricots and lemons and in aspartame, the sugar substitute. It's one of the reasons chocolate provides a lift.

enzymes that perform more than 700 separate activities. 100,000 enzyme particles alone can be found in a single drop of blood.)

Sprouts—A Top Source of Fat-Free Protein

The process of sprouting makes protein more readily available as well. Protein is something else you may be shorting yourself on if you're reducing your fat intake. (Fat and protein go together in nine out of 10 foods.) Without enough protein you go to pot. A deficiency can cause a decrease in heart, lung, liver and kidney functions. Effects show up in skin, bone and muscles where over 60 percent of your body's protein is stored. The protein content of sprouts used in dried form[16] compares favorably to egg and meat protein, and then some, say researchers Jeffrey Bland, Ph.D. and Barbara Berquist. Even better, sprouts supply lecithin, the magic substance in soybeans that speeds up fat breakdown, digestion and cholesterol reduction and spares you unwanted calories.

The next best thing about sprouts is their turnover value. Sprouts can be converted into an alternative to almost any sweetener you eat and think you can't live without—such as white sugar, for instance (see *One Ingredient Bread*, page 79 or baked goods).

There are countless seeds you can sprout. Here's a useful rule of thumb: 1 pound of seed yield between 6 and 8 pounds of sprouts. The table below shows a few good ones for starters.

Note: If you want sprouts' vitamins without sprouting, buy dehydrated wheat and dried barley leaf powder, sold as wheat grass tablets and powder, and Green Magma powder and tablets (see *Sources*.) Both provide most of the chlorophyll, protein, calcium, fiber, vitamin A and antioxidants you get from sprouts, and they're organically grown to boot. They're also useful as a sprinkle seasoning or a base for juices and soups. You can bury seeds to sprout singly, buy assorted and ready-to-eat sprouts or grow your own.

	Amount of Seed (for Quart Size Jar)	Soaking Time (Hrs)	Sprouting Time (Days)	Length at Harvest (Inches)
Alfalfa*	2½ T	8	4–6	1½–2
Clover*	2½ T	8	4–6	1½–2
Garbanzo Bean (chickpea)	1 C	14	3	½
Lentil	¾ C	10	2–3	¼–½
Mung Bean	⅓ cup	16	2–5	1–3

---

[16]How to use sprouts in dried form? See Wholewheat Sweetener recipe (page 116).

	Amount of Seed for Quart Jar	Soaking Time	Sprouting Time	Length at Harvest
Radish*	3 T	10	4–5	1–2
Rye, whole berries	1 C	12	2–3	1
Soybean	¾ C	12	3–4	½–2
Sunflower*	1 C	10	2–5	¼–½
Wheat	1 C	12	2–3	1–1½

Key

*Sprouts that sprout leaves. After day one, put them near a window so leaves can develop chlorophyll.
C = cup
T = tablespoon
Information courtesy of *The Sproutletter* (see *Sources*).

How to Grow Your Own Sprouts

1. Use a large wide-mouth container such as a 1-quart Mason jar plus a square of cheesecloth, gauze, netting or nylon to cover the jar opening. Put ¼ to ½ cup of dry seeds into jar. (A good beginner's mixture? Three teaspoons alfalfa plus 5 teaspoons of lentils. A few mung beans or whole wheat may be added.)

2. Fill jar half-full with lukewarm water. After eight hours, agitate jar and fasten netting in place with a rubberband and pour off soaking water. Place jar on its side in a warm, dark spot in the kitchen. Rinse and drain seeds twice a day with tepid water without removing netting. After two days place container in indirect sunlight to increase chlorophyll content. If you are sprouting a seed that grows leaves (see list), place in indirect sunlight.

3. Most seeds sprout in three to five days. When the "tails" are about twice as long as the seed itself, they are ready to eat. For maximum nutrition eat the whole sprout, eat it raw and eat it soon.

4. Do not freeze sprouts. Nutritional value lies in their freshness. Instead, cover any surplus with cold water and refrigerate for no more than four days.

5. Use only chemically untreated and certified edible seeds. Avoid water with fluorine or chlorine or similar chemicals. These may sterilize the seed's embryo and prevent germination.

To learn more about the ABC's of sprouting everything from Amaranth to Quinoa, write: Hippocrates Health Institute, 25 Exeter Street, Boston, MA 02116, or The Sproutletter Institute, P.O. Box 62, Ashland, OR 97520.

Sources of stay-young sprouts

• Fresh sprouts (sold singly and in mixtures at produce sections).

• Dried sprouts (sold as diastolic malt powder [a bread leavener]) available from Ross Industries, Box 2696, Wichita, KS 67201.

• Seeds to sprout (see *Sources*).

• Sprouted breads such as Essene.

• Freeze-dried sprouts (health food stores).

HONEY, POLLEN, PROPOLIS

Three Sweet-Tooth Foods That Help You Stay Young

In the Soviet Union, when biologist and experimental botanist of the Longevity Institute of the USSR, Dr. Nicolai Tsitsin, sent out letters to more than 200 residents who claimed to be more than 100 years old, he asked three questions: What was their age, occupation and principal food? Of the 150 responses, a large number of the long-lifers reported beekeeping as their profession and bee pollen as a daily staple.

Even if you don't keep bees, you can keep bee pollen in your pantry, and you should, along with other bee-based foods such as bee propolis (an antibiotic), royal jelly (a beauty aid) and honey. There is no sweeter, safer way to slow the aging process.

Pollen might turn you into a post-30's tower of power—President Reagan takes it daily. So does Noel Johnson, 82-year-old World Senior Boxing Champion, lecturer, and the oldest living finisher of the 1979 New York City Marathon, who says he made the use of bee pollen the essential facet of his nutrition program. "I believe I derive special nutrients from bee pollen which produced the energy I needed for the Pikes Peak Marathon and other events . . ."

Use Pollen as a Rejuvenator

Pollen may not be perfect but it's a good addition to any life-extension pantry. The British Sports Council has recorded increases in strength, stamina and endurance as great as 40 to 50 percent in measured performance after a period of pollen therapy. According to the Institute of Bee Culture in Paris, which has conducted double-blind studies and research into the benefits of bee pollen, it has been used successfully in weight loss, fighting insomnia, virus infections, even anemia and correcting faulty digestion. Pollen is a good energizer (it's 40 percent natural sugar in the form of fructose and glucose). And according to the director of the Bee Laboratory at the U.S. Department of Agriculture Research Center in Beltsville, Maryland, the protein content of pollen ranges from 5 to 28 percent. (By comparison, tofu has 46 percent protein; raw soybean, 38 percent; pumpkin seeds have 29 percent; brewer's yeast, 39 percent and round steak is 20 percent.)

Six Amazing Reasons Pollen Makes You Look and Feel Younger

Pollen is a good source of nucleic acids which explains its ability to harmonize body functions, build strength, normalize weight and soothe nerves. Pollen even builds red corpuscles and fights cancer. Increases in quantity of red corpuscles by 25 to 30 percent with an increase in hemoglobin count of 15 percent have been commonly recorded. And according to New York Cancer Research, beekeepers as a group,[17] have the lowest incidence of cancer of all occupations the NCR has monitored. Dr. George E. Berkey, Boston State College, reported on a French study of the deaths of 1,000 beekeepers that showed only one death from cancer. A control group of non-beekeeping French farmers showed a fatal cancer rate 100 times higher.

Propolis—Nature's Wonder Drug

However you take it, stick with it and give it time. Bee pollen's benefits, say experts, are progressive and gradual.

Another A-1 bee food is propolis, a brownish, resinous substance gathered by bees from the leaf buds or bark of trees. They add a glandular secretion to this juice or sap and use it like cement to seal and tighten the hive and—of more interest to us—also to protect themselves from bacterial and viral infections. The word "propolis" comes from the Greek, meaning "before a city," because the bees deposit propolis near the opening of the hive to sterilize anything entering it.

It has been reported that an animal embalmed in propolis will remain intact without decomposing for five to six years. In the human term, propolis has been found to promote many sorts of healing, especially of disorders involving infections. The Greek physician Hippocrates, called the "father of medicine," prescribed propolis as far back as 400 B.C. to help heal sores, ulcers and wounds. It was used to speed healing of wounds and to disinfect surgical instruments in many wars, including World War II.

Studies conducted in Yugoslavia during an influenza epidemic, compared one group of nursing students who took propolis daily with another control group who did not. Two and a half times more people in the control group got the flu. A study in Austria found the 90 percent of 108 patients hospitalized with ulcers who were given propolis were free of symptoms after two weeks, compared to 55 percent of the 185 patients treated conventionally.

---

[17]The United States has 2,700 commercial beekeepers and 4 million hobbyists.

Seven Ways to Use Propolis Regularly

Propolis is effective as preventive medicine to build up resistance to infection, skin problems and sore gums and as a natural medicine for colds and other illnesses for which manmade antibiotics are ordinarily prescribed. (Propolis is a natural antibiotic but has not been found to have the harmful side effects which sometimes accompany manmade antibiotics.) You can buy propolis in the form of capsules, powders, tablets, tinctures, lozenges and even chips for chewing. It is also used in beauty products and toothpastes.

Do You Know What Famous First Family Uses Propolis Daily?

As for royal jelly? What's good enough for Britain's entire royal family (who reportedly start their day with this life-extension stuff) should be good enough for you. According to French nutritionist Alain Caillas, royal jelly has been successfully used to treat Parkinson's Disease, heart and liver ailments, arthritis and ulcers. True royal jelly is sold in airtight capsules or freeze-dried tablets, with or without pollen.

Honey—Keep It in Your Medicine Cabinet

Pure honey can be a honey of a health food, too, even if too few of us eat it.[18] Bees have been around 55 to 60 million years before man. The hive is as old as the hills. Twenty-thousand-year-old drawings in Spanish caves depict a man climbing cliffs to raid hives. The Neolithic lake dwellers in Switzerland made vessels for straining honey, and honey is mentioned hundreds of times in the Bible. Egyptians used honey as a surgical dressing, ancient Hebrews valued it as a healing agent for ulcerated wounds and much of Europe used it for deep cuts and skin inflammations during the Middle Ages.

Six Special Benefits Honey Supplies

A Slavic treatment for sleeplessness uses a combination of two tablespoons of honey with the juice of a lemon and an orange. The ancient Chinese used honey and herbs to treat a weak heart, and Hungarian folk remedies include honey poultices for gout-inflamed feet. German studies suggest honey helps heal ulcers. The enzymes in honey also enhance the digestive processes. Honey is easily assimilated and does not remain in the stomach or promote irritation of the lining and is handled far better by the kidneys than sugar. It even has a mild laxative effect.

---

[18]Less than 20 percent of the population ever eats honey, says the USDA.

Honey vs. Sugar: Important Facts

Honey contains small amounts of potassium, chloride, sulphur, sodium, phosphorus, magnesium, silica, iron, copper and manganese, in addition to enzymes, amino acids, minute quantities of the B vitamins and a trace of vitamin C. Honey with pollen residue supplies life-lengthening nucleic acids as well.

But more important than what it *does* do, is what it doesn't do. Unlike sugar, honey has no potential for causing cancer. Stephen Seely of the University of Manchester in England and Dr. D. F. Horrobin of Nova Scotia investigated the amount of sugar eaten in 20 countries and compared figures with the incidence of breast cancer in these same countries. Results? The countries with the most breast cancer were the countries with the highest consumption of sugar—England, Netherlands, then Ireland, Canada and Denmark. Countries with the lowest consumption of sugar and of breast cancer were Italy, Yugoslavia, Spain, Portugal and Japan. In Japan, the average consumption of sugar and sugary foods is only 60 grams a day—15 teaspoons. In the United States, the average American consumes 36 teaspoons.

The researchers say sugar causes insulin to be over-secreted by the pancreas, and then it is poured into the bloodstream. This state seems to act on low-priority tissues as a mild carcinogen (cancer-causer). The human breast is an organ of "low priority."

Tips on Shopping for Honey

Honey isn't the real thing if it's pollen-free or over-processed. If honey has been heated and filtered (to remove pollen which causes cloudiness), what's left is mostly sugar. Commercial packers heat honey to approximately 150°F so it can be pumped easily through their system of filters, producing an end product with a longer shelf life but lower nutritional value, because the pollen in the honey is what contributes most of the nutrients. The best honey is darker with a tendency to crystallize on the shelf, the label comes with a flower source, and it is sold at health food stores or bought directly from a roadside stand run by a beekeeper.

Top sources of life-extending bee foods

- Raw honeycomb supplies bioflavonoids (vitamin P)
- Raw liquid honey
- Desserts and snacks made with honey
- Bee pollen granules, powders, tablets or liquid
- Bee pollen desserts and candies
- Royal jelly supplements
- Beauty aids made with royal jelly

- Propolis tincture
- Propolis powder
- Propolis lozenges and chips
- Propolis/pollen capsules and candies
- Pollen-propolis nutritional supplements

Note: According to Dr. Sheldon Reiser, chief of the Carbohydrate Nutrition Laboratory, Agriculture Research Center of the U.S. Department of Agriculture, "Feeding rats sugar rather than starch, vegetables, grains, nuts, etc. increases the rate of absorption of sugars through the intestines, producing raised levels of insulin and increased activity of those body enzymes which change carbohydrate to fat. Without exception, the rats on the high-sugar diets developed pre-diabetic symptoms, relating to disorders of blood sugar and blood fats." Sugar may even be a carcinogen (see *Anti-Aging Ingredients: Honey*, page 65).

In short, less sugar means greater health. So what *do* you use to sweeten your unfrosted, live-longer flakes? Your options? A do-no-evil sweetener or a do-it-yourself sugar is best. Store-bought choices—all of which supply iron, calcium and B vitamins—include natural, unprocessed honey (with the comb intact for the most nutrients), maple syrup and maple syrup "sprinkles," sorghum syrup, rice syrups, date "sugar" and barley malt granules or liquid sweetener, unsulphured molasses, and for an occasional treat "real" cane sugar (see *Sources*) which gives you almost half your calcium for the day in a 4-ounce helping.

Pass up sugar substitutes of all kinds. Saccharin is a carcinogen which actually increases rather than depresses appetite in many dieters, and commercial aspartame has an adverse effect on brain chemistry. As for most of the fructose (fruit sugar) sold, the Washington, D.C.-based Center for Science in the Public Interest advises it's highly refined from corn not fruit and poses the same health hazards as refined sugar.

FIVE LIFE-EXTENSION PROGRAMS: DAILY MENUS

Now that you know *what* to eat, how do you make a meal of it? Here are four plans. They don't work miracles, but they work. The magic lies in the moderation. The menus are planned to keep you underfed, optimally nourished and feeling like 20 at 50. Each day supplies roughly 1500 to 1800 calories—plan 4 has even less if that's what you need more of—enough to fuel a 150-pound middle-aged male or a 120-pound female (add or subtract food and calories if you're neither). Each makes maximum use of age-proof ingredients and nutrients. And if you use the *real* foods it calls for, you'll feel satisfied, low as that calorie intake sounds.

As a bonus, each day's menus follow the guidelines set by the American Health Foundation and the Duke University "Dupac Diet' (preventive approach to cardiovascular disease which emphasizes high-complex carbohydrates with little meat), considered the best diet available for preventing heart disease, the country's number-one killer. They supply less than 2 grams of sodium and less than 25 grams of fat[19] that experts recommend for health and long life. If you're faithful, you should be thinner in a month no matter which one of these no-room-for-improvement, live-longer diets you decide to take seriously.

Last, but not least—to help you digest your food and food supplements well and get more from them—invest in a good enzymatic digestive aid. The best kinds are formulated in two layers so their gentle but effective action works twice. The pepsin and papain in the outer layer work to aid the digestive process in your stomach, and the enzymatic action helps release inner corn ingredients into your intestines. One or two tablets with meals helps digestion of starches, proteins and fats, and prevents heartburn and gas.

Plan I

Directions: Here's an easy approach to live-longer meal plans. If you never know what your day or your fridge has in store for you, it's for you. Just eat at least two portions from List A, three from B, two from C and two from D. Choose any of the portions you like and eat them at any meal. Just be sure to get the total of nine portions to get in your total life-extending nutrition for the day. Season with a salt substitute, pepper, or lemon juice where desired.

Column A (protein)[20]	*Column B (vegetables)*
chicken (skinned white meat) (3–4 oz.)	asparagus (8 stalks)
codfish (3–4 oz.)	string beans (½ cup)
tempeh or tofu (3–4 oz.)	dried beans (½ cup)
egg (1)	broccoli (½ cup)
flounder or sole (3–4 oz.)	cabbage (½ cup)
halibut or salmon (4–5 oz.)*	carrots (½ cup)
sardines (¾ oz.)*	cauliflower (½ cup)
scallops (4 oz.)	celery (4 stalks)
tuna (3 oz., water-packed, drained)	cucumber (1 medium)
turkey (2 oz. skinned white meat)	eggplant (½ cup)
skim milk (1 cup)	baked potato (1 small)
*With bones	green or red bell pepper (½ cup)
	lettuces (1 cup any type)

---

[19]How to figure your fat intake? See *Diet Tips* (pages 14–18).
[20]Use salt-reduced when available.

buttermilk or acidophilus milk (4 oz.)

yogurt or kefir (4 oz.)

low-calorie cottage cheese or farmer's cheese (3 oz.)

hamburger (4 oz. lean)

hard cheese (1 oz.)

dark, leafy greens (1 cup any type)

mushrooms (½ cup, cooked)

green onions (4)

sprouts (½ cup)

radishes (10)

sauerkraut (½ cup)

spinach (½ cup)

squash (½ cup)

tomato (1 medium, raw)

green or yellow zucchini (½ cup)

watercress (½ cup)

vinegar (any amount)

diet dressing (1 teaspoon)

Column C (breads and cereals)[20]

whole-wheat bagel (1)

whole-grain English muffin (½)

whole-grain hard roll, biscuit or bun (half)

whole-grain melba toast (3 sl.)

bread (thin sliced rye, whole wheat, pumpernickel)

hot cereal (Wheatena, 7 grain, buckwheat, oatmeal, etc.) (½ cup)

cold cereal, sugar-free (i.e., shredded wheat) (½ cup)

sweet potato (½ cup)

whole-wheat or rye crackers (4–5)

soy or lima beans (½ cup)

corn or brown rice (½ cup)

Column D (fruits and juices)[20]

apple or plum (1 medium)

apricots (2) or peach (1)

bananas (1 medium)

cantaloupe or other melon (half)

cherries (½ cup)

dates (1)

figs (4 oz.)

fruit cocktail, sugar-free (3 oz.)

grapefruit or other citrus fruit (½ medium)

grapes (½ cup)

mango or papaya (4 oz.)

nectarine (1 small)

orange (1 medium)

sliced pineapple (4 oz.)

prunes (2 small)

raspberries, blueberries or strawberries (½ cup)

tangerine (1 medium) or kiwi fruit (2)

watermelon (1 small wedge)

Juices (3 oz. unsweetened)

apple cider

cranberry

cherry

grape (white or purple)
orange
pineapple
grapefruit
prune
tomato
V-8
Fruit-juice "popsicles" (sugar-
    free) count as 2 servings

Plan II

If your meals are giving you a square deal nutritionally, you can define them by all the things they *don't* contain—such as saturated fat, refined sugar, salt and empty calories.

This meal plan is free of all these aging-additives and provides a more detailed approach to longevity eating. It's even a 1,500-calorie-a-day reducing diet that doesn't look like one because although it *cuts* portions, it *increases* your food choices, thereby improving overall nutritional benefit. The calories have been pre-counted for you each day.

Day one

Breakfast

1 raisin bran muffin, spread with 2 tablespoons farmer's cheese,
    or low-fat cream cheese
1 vitamin C croissant[21] with two 10-calorie curls of unsalted
    butter (page 103)
Café au lait (4 oz. decaf coffee prepared with skim milk plus
    cinnamon or nutmeg)

Lunch

Tossed salad: salad greens, carrots, green pepper, tomato,
    sprouts with 2 oz. low-fat shredded cheese, 1 teaspoon lemon
    juice, salt substitute
1 cup True Blue greens[21] with self-dressing
2 sesame breadsticks or crackers
8 oz. glass of sparkling mineral water on the rocks, or
1 glass of Iced Atomic Tea[21]

Snack

3 oz. raw mixed nuts, or

---

[21]See recipe.

1 tablespoon nut butter spread (peanut, cashew, walnut, etc.) on a sliced, fresh apple, or

2 pieces Seeds of Health Salami[21] with Stay-Young Herbal Tea[21] or Live-Longer Ginseng Milkshake[21]

Dinner

4 oz. baked or broiled lean fish (sole, flounder, cod, etc.) with ½ cup sliced mushrooms and 1 tablespoon grated parmesan cheese, or

2 Red Pepper Pancakes[21] with alfalfa sprouts

6 oz. chilled orange, pineapple or papaya juice

½ cup fresh fruit cocktail (cantaloupe, oranges, red and green grapes), or

1 Vitamin P Parfait[21]

Day two

Breakfast

½ whole-wheat English muffin, 1 poached or coddled egg, 1 teaspoon salt-free butter or 1 teaspoon olive oil

Tea au lait (4 oz. decaf with skim milk and cinnamon)

Lunch

Tuna curry pita: wholewheat pita filled with 2½ oz. drained water-packed tuna, 1 tablespoon raisins, 1 small apple, grated, 1 teaspoon mayo, ⅛ teaspoon curry powder plus ½ cup lettuce and tomato, diced.

1 8-oz. glass of iced herb tea

1 sugar-free frozen juice bar

Snack

2 small sugar-free gingersnaps

6 oz. buttermilk, or Calcium Sip[21]

Dinner

3 oz. tofu or 3 oz. tempeh, baked or broiled with 1 teaspoon low-sodium soy sauce and 1 teaspoon safflower oil

Medium baked potato with 2 tablespoons yogurt, 2 tablespoons chives

½ cup steamed zucchini and/or yellow squash

1 6-oz. grape juice spritzer (3 oz. each white grape juice and sparkling water)

½ fresh papaya with toasted wheat germ or bran

Day three

Breakfast

> 1 cup whole-grain hot cereal with 2 chopped apricots and ¼ cup skim milk, or
> 1 cup Beta-Carotene Baked endive[21]
> 4 oz. any fresh, unsweetened fruit juice

Lunch

> 1 slice natural mushroom/green pepper/cheese pizza, or
> 1 square Longevity Loaf #1[21]
> 1 large bunch fresh grapes

Snack

> Life Extension Smoothie (whip ½ cup plain yogurt ½ small banana and ½ cup apple juice in blender)

Dinner

> *Take-Out Chinese* (specify no salt, no monosodium glutamate)
> 1 cup wonton soup
> 1½ cup mixed seafood with Chinese vegetables
> ½ cup rice
> 2 fortune cookies
> *Add at Home*:
> 1 orange or tangerine, sectioned, sprinkled with maple syrup sprinkles
> 1 cup decaf or herb tea

Day four

Breakfast

> 1 cup shredded wheat, or
> 1 vitamin C croissant[21]
> ½ cup frozen blueberries, thawed or ½ cup fresh
> 1 cup skim milk or buttermilk or sweet acidophilus milk

Lunch

> Egg or Tofu Club Salad: 2 chopped eggs or 1 square tofu, diced, ¼ cup chopped celery, 2 tablespoons yogurt or fat-reduced mayonnaise on 3 slices of toasted, seeded natural rye or pumpernickel
> Orange-Plus Shake: ¾ cup plain, lowfat yogurt blended with ½ cup unsweetened pineapple juice

---

[21]See recipe.

Snack

> 1 cup air-popped popcorn with grated cheese, or
> 1 frozen fruit juice bar, or
> 1 cup 50-Plus Pudding[21]

Dinner

> Sea Stirfry: 10 small cooked shrimp, 1 cup cooked brown rice or
>   steamed buckwheat (kasha), or
> Longevity Loaf #2[21]
> ½ cup V-8 or tomato juice or 1 cup alcohol-free wine
> 1 cup steamed carrots, or 1 ear fresh corn steamed
> 1 cup diced tropical fruit (papaya, mango, prickly pear, etc.) or 1
>   small peach, pear or kiwi fruit

• Now what? Repeat the menus—but with different food combinations. Possible combinations are endless, more if you really make use of the recipes in this book and use your imagination.

Here's how and why the plan works:

• Fuel yourself with three-meals-plus-snacks a day, but keep portion sizes small. In other words, if you can't eat light, eat half. This will make a weight maintenance pattern easier later on.

• Cut back on fatty foods (whole milk, rice, cheese, ice cream), and eliminate red meat, using leaner, skinless poultry, fish and meat substitutes.

• Fill up on fiber-rich grains, fruits, vegetables.

• Include one serving each of proteins, grains and vegetables to guarantee satisfaction of your need for nutrients, taste and texture.

• Snack on fruits—have two or more servings a day.

Plan III

Here's another get-young, stay-young formula that doesn't even call for a measuring cup, let alone a head for calories. The following provides all the age-proofing nutrients you need, especially the nucleic acids complex. It raises energy levels and lowers cholesterol, and it's what put no-aging diet expert Dr. Benjamin S. Frank on the map.

1. Eat seafood seven times a week. Four of these seafood meals can be a 3- or 4-ounce can of small sardines (not the big ones in the oval cans but the small ones, usually from Portugal; pour off any oil from the sardines to save fat and calories). Have salmon once, shrimp once and any other kind of fish or sea vegetables once. Lobsters, clams, crabs, anchovies and oysters are also rich in sardines' star nutrient—nucleic acids—and any of these can be served once a week.

2. Have soybeans, peas, lentils or lima beans once or twice a week.

3. Serve liver once a week.

4. Eat beets three times a week (beet juice and borsht are valuable, too). Beets contain an amino acid which helps build nucleic acid, and reportedly improves general brain function.

5. Add two of the following each day to meals: cauliflower, celery, mushrooms, sprouts, onions, radishes, asparagus, spinach, scallions.

6. One or 2 ounces of raw nuts or seeds or sprouts a day.

7. Two glasses of skim milk, yogurt or buttermilk every day.

8. One to two glasses of fresh fruit or vegetable juice once daily.

9. Three or four glasses of pure-as-possible water every day. Buy bottled if you aren't sure what's running from your tap.

10. Take a good name-brand, high-potency multivitamin every day plus any extra life-extending nutrients you are using.

Plan IV

Another way to put longevity on the menu is to eat the way three of the world's seniors-who-look-like-juniors do—

	Dietary Staple (daily)
Hunza Valley, Pakistan (many between 90 and 100 years) . . . 1,923 calories daily	Apricots, mulberries Chapati bread Raw lettuce, onions and root vegetables Goats' milk and fresh butter (small amounts)
Abkhazia, Caucasus, U.S.S.R. (1 out of 300 is over 100 years) . . . 1,700–1,900 calories daily	Vegetables (70% of total calories) Low-fat cheese and buttermilk Fruit (especially grapes) Chicken, beef, goat, pork (limited) Cornmeal bread Red pepper, black pepper, garlic Locally pressed, dry red wine (daily in moderate amounts) Lean meat only a few times a year
Vilcabamba, Ecuador (total absence of heart disease and other serious ailments) . . . 1,200 calories daily	Corn and other whole grains Yucca root (available at U.S. health food stores) Dried beans

Potatoes
Fruit (especially banana)
Bean soups with homemade
white cheese

Plan V

Crash diets are hazardous and aging. But here's a fast and healthy 800-calorie-a-day diet plan that won't endanger your health or your youth potential. It uses fresh fruits to produce a look-younger/feel-younger effect.

Directions: Use it for no more than three days at a time or more than once a month and drink plenty of water. Between times, switch to one of the other diet plans in this book. Each recipe below equals one mini-meal. Feel free to reverse the order of the menus (variations apply to brown-baggers):

Meal One

Two-Fruit Frappe: Combine ½ cup fresh or carton orange juice in the blender with 4 fresh or frozen strawberries and 2–3 crushed ice cubes. Blend until frothy. 70 calories.

Variations: Have Meal Two in place of Meal One and in place of Meal Two, have a desktop snack of fresh berries with a 4-ounce carton on the side.

Meal Two

Fluffernutter Shake: Combine in a blender or food processor ¾ cup unsweetened, crushed pineapple, ½ small banana, ¼ cup cracker ice and 1½ teaspoons peanut butter; blend until frothy. 88 calories.

Meal Three

Blender Gazpacho: Put all these in blender: ½ cup canned plum tomatoes, drained, or 1 ripe tomato, chopped, ¼ diced small cucumber, 1 tablespoon minced bell pepper, 1 tablespoon chopped onion, 2 teaspoons lemon juice, ¼ teaspoon dried oregano, dash of hot pepper sauce; blend until smooth. Chill and serve in a bowl topped with 1 teaspoon each minced parsley.

Variation: Make soup the night before and tote (with lo-cal crackers) in a thermos.

Meal Four

Tangerine Crush: Juice of 1 small, peeled tangerine (by hand or electric juicer) and ½ small, peeled grapefruit (or substitute ¼ cup presqueezed, store-bought orange juice and ½ cup store-brought grapefruit juice); combine juices with 2–3 cracked ice cubes in a blender. Whip to a froth. 73 calories.

Variation: Eat the tangerine and drink a 4-ounce can or bottle of grapefruit juice.

Meal Five

6 O'Clock Smoothie: Combine in blender ½ cup fresh or unsweetened frozen blueberries, ½ cup unsweetened frozen peach slices, ¼ small frozen banana, sliced, 1 teaspoon wheat germ and 5 cracked ice cubes; blend until smooth and frothy. Serve with 1 tablespoon mixed almonds and sunflower seeds on the side. 160 calories.

Meal Six

Nightcap Nog: Puree ¼ small, peeled and frozen banana, ¼ cup skim milk, 1½ teaspoons nut butter, 1 teaspoon raisins, 5 crushed ice cubes; blend until smooth. Drink with a sprinkle of nutmeg. 95 calories.

RECIPES FOR A LONGER LIFE

LIVE-LONGER BENEFITS: INGREDIENTS

1. Benefits heart and circulation, blood pressure.
2. Provides cancer protection.
3. Aids weight control.
4. Improves resistance and immunity.
5. Rejuvenates nervous system and improves stress tolerance.
6. Improves energy levels.
7. Maintains healthy bones and teeth, prevents loss of bone, promotes dental health.

Every recipe in this book offers time-fighting benefits as documented by such organizations as the National Institute of Health, the American Cancer Society and the American Herb Trade Association. To find the specific benefits a recipe offers, check out the numbers which correspond to the above chart.

BREADS/BREAKFAST

First things first. That means good bread and a better breakfast. If you're anything like the rest of us, it's probably time to change your doughnut-dunkin' ways.

According to a recent survey—on any given day—nearly half of America's prime-of-life population passes up breakfast, often trying to lose weight. Don't! Skipping or skimping on breakfast does not make you thinner faster. Meal-skippers in general are *more* likely to be obese than those who eat three meals a day. A study of college women showed that those who skip breakfast do more all-day snacking than those who eat breakfast. Another risk associated with skipping breakfast is that you're likely to miss important longevity nutrients, including vitamin C, riboflavin and calcium. Most of us, surveys say, don't get enough of these in the two meals that remain.

Lecithins (whole-wheat crackers)

• Preheat oven to 425°.
• Combine 2 cups whole-wheat flour and 1½ teaspoons *Life Extension Salt* (page 106). With a fork, stir in ½ cup plus 2 tablespoons water and 5 tablespoons corn or olive oil until blended. Turn dough onto a lightly floured board sprinkled with 5 tablespoons lecithin granules and knead until smooth, about 10 minutes. Pinch off 16 small rolls of dough. Roll thin. Flatten with tines of a fork as you would peanut butter cookies. Sprinkle with dried onion or green pepper flakes, sesame or poppy seeds and bake until golden. Cool on a cake rack.

Variation #1:

Lecithins (rye crackers)

• Pre-heat oven to 425°
• Combine 1 cup rye flour with 1 cup all-purpose flour (unsifted), 1 teaspoon natural sugar and ½ teaspoon *Life Extension Salt* (page 106). With a fork, stir in ½ cup warm water or tea and 5 tablespoons melted, unsalted butter until blended. Add more water if needed. Turn dough onto a lightly floured board sprinkled with 5 tablespoons lecithin granules and knead until smooth, about 10 minutes. Cool as directed above.

Variation #2:
For crust-not-crackers—roll out either dough, and press into greased pie pan, thin, flute edges. Bake 10 minutes at 350°. Cook and fill or add any fruit or vegetable filling first, and then bake 50 minutes at 350°.
Uses: A crunch munch, a chip dip or see variation#2 above.
Stay Young Note: If you're crackers for crackers, one reason to bake them, not buy them is their sodium content. Here's how salty America's three favorites are, per ounce: Ritz (290 mg.); Triscuits (210); Saltines (345).
Supplies: LONGEVITY BENEFITS *1, 3, 6, 8.*

One-ingredient bread (yeast and flour-free)

1–1½ cups whole-wheat berries

• Soak berries in water overnight then drain and sprout.
• After three days when shoots appear, rinse well and pulverize in a blender (dough will be tacky). Knead. (Oil your hands if mixture is too sticky.)
• Knead dough ten minutes until you have a pliable dough ball. The gluten in the sprouts will develop and hold the dough together, but it won't be as "elastic" as regular bread dough.
• Form into a loaf shape, and place on oiled baking sheet.
• Bake in 350° oven for ten minutes until baked all the way through and brown on top. Use a wet knife with a serrated blade to slice.

About two dozen slices.
Uses: A good breakfast bread—ground sprouts are a concentrated source of grain sugar energy. Or serve as a low-calorie fruit-cake substitute.
Variations: Substitute a whole-grain such as rye, unhulled oats, barley, whole brown rice or triticale (rye-wheat hybrid) etc., in place of wheat; add ½ cup of any finely diced dry fruit or raw seeds before you knead.
Stay Young Note: When grains sprout, the fattening starch they contain turns into unfattening protein. Sprouting also increases sweetness,

says the Hippocrates Health Institute of Boston. Sprouted breads are better tolerated and digested by the grain- and flour-sensitive, and this bread is safe for mold allergy sufferers because it's yeast-free.

Life-extension muffins (the Breakfast Danish alternative)

2 oz. unsalted butter

4 tablespoons date "sugar" or maple sugar plus 3 tablespoons black-strap molasses

¼ cup mashed banana

2 eggs, beaten

1 cup buttermilk

2 cups bran (oat, wheat, rice or corn) soaked in ½ cup hot water or herb tea

½ cup dried chopped dates or raisins

1 cup stoneground whole-wheat pastry flour

1 tablespoon soy flour, grits or meal, or soy lecithin granules

¾ teaspoon baking soda.

- In a large bowl, cream butter, "sugar," banana, molasses.
- Add eggs to buttermilk or yogurt and stir. Add dried fruits and stir well to combine.
- Sift dry ingredients together and add to wet ingredients. Spoon batter into wells of a well-greased mini-cupcake tin. Bake in greased cupcake tins at 375° for 15 minutes, or bake all the batter as a cake in a 8¼ × 8" pan.

Makes a dozen 125-calorie meal-in-a-bite buns.

Uses: As a two-bite breakfast, a snack or cupcake alternative.

Variations: Use yogurt, kefir or blender-whipped tofu in place of buttermilk; use 2 tablespoons sweet miso paste or 2 tablespoons of honey in place of molasses.

Stay Young Note: Have you exercised your way to one more 130-calorie, guilt-free bun? Here's how to tell: Walking a mile in 20 minutes burns 235–285 calories if you weigh 120 pounds, 270–330 calories if you weigh 150 pounds, 285–335 calories if you weigh 175 pounds. Riding a motorcycle burns three times as many calories per minute as sleeping.

Supplies: LONGEVITY BENEFITS *1, 5, 6, 8.*

40-plus rye crisps (wheat-free thins)

1½ cups rye flour

1 teaspoon each caraway and sesame seed

1 teaspoon low-sodium baking powder

4 tablespoons oil or butter

4 tablespoons water or herb tea

• Sift flour and baking powder. Cut in butter or oil plus enough water to make a stiff dough. Roll out on floured board. Sprinkle with seed. Score. Bake 10–15 minutes at 400°, or until brown. Cool on cake rack.

Uses: To use as a pie shell—after rolling out, press into a greased 9″ pie tin, pick with a fork, fill and bake. Or wrap and freeze until needed.

Variations: Substitute corn meal or barley flour for rye.

Stay Young Note: Are you a sugarholic? To reduce the urge to indulge, take a tip from the Orientals and add a pinch of sugar to your main dish.

Supplies: LONGEVITY BENEFITS *1, 6, 8.*

SALADS/SOUPS

Toss a good salad and you can stop right there. Salads can help you preserve what you've got and even improve on it. With the right add-ins, they make complete meals. And it's just as easy to make your own life-extension pot boilers.

Here are some go-for-broke salads and soups that make complete live-longer meals or make life-extending meals complete.

Age-proof escarole salad

1 head escarole (about ¾ lb.)

1 head red leaf or romaine lettuce (about ½ lb.)

1 tablespoon Dijon or Dijon-style mustard

2 tablespoons red-wine vinegar

1 teaspoon finely minced garlic

Freshly ground pepper to taste

6 tablespoons olive oil

• Cut away and discard the core from each head of lettuce. Rinse and pat or spin-dry the leaves. Cut the leaves into bite-size pieces, and place in salad bowl.

• Put the mustard, vinegar, garlic and pepper in a mixing bowl; gradually add oil and stir well using a wire whisk.

• Spoon dressing over greens. Toss to blend well.

Serves 4 to 6.

Uses: A first course or a high-fiber dessert for sweets-abstainers.

Variations: To make a "whole meal" escarole salad, add 1 cup cooked tempeh, tofu or sea vegetables.

Stay Young Note: Why use escarole and not iceberg? It's higher in vitamin A, three times richer in calcium and, as a bonus, you get more vitamin C. Even better, add a little lemony-flavored sorrel. This French lettuce/herb supplies more vitamin A (10,240 I.U.) than any longevity green, including parsley, basil or beet greens. Its lemon flavor and taste marries well with onion and tomatoes.

• Supplies LONGEVITY BENEFITS *2, 3, 4, 5, 7, 8.*

Mock crabmeat salad

2 cups raw shredded parsnips

1 cup finely sliced celery or celery root

1 tablespoon chopped pimento or raw red bell pepper

½ cup quartered ripe olives or ¼ cup bottled green peppercorns

½ cup low-sodium mayonnaise

1 tablespoon lemon juice

2 teaspoons finely sliced green onions or garlic greens

¾ teaspoon kelp powder or any salt substitute (page 106)

Fresh ground black or white pepper to taste

• Mix the first 4 ingredients.
• Blend in mayonnaise, lemon juice, onion and seasonings.
• Combine all ingredients and mound on a bed of dark greens (kale, collard, spinach). *Optional*: A handful of cold, stir-fried sea vegetables such as hizichi adds color, trace minerals and vitamin A.

Serves 4.

Uses: Serves as a first course or add cubes of cooked tofu or tempeh for a whole meal salad.

Variations: Substitute water chestnuts, chayote squash or jicama for celery (see note below).

Stay Young Note: According to Dr. Jordon Fink, chief of the allergy section of the Medical College of Wisconsin, in three reported cases in Milwaukee, celery-munchers who exercised vigorously after eating, suffered a severe allergic reaction. One case progressed to a condition of shock in which the victim's circulatory system caused the stricken celery-eater to collapse into unconsciousness. The condition known as food-dependent exercise-induced anaphylaxis, is an extreme allergic reaction that can be fatal in some cases if untreated, says the *British Medical Journal.* In each of the three cases, the victims, two tennis players and a jogger, suffered shortness of breath, profuse sweating, weakness and abdominal cramps. For the non-sensitive, celery contributes fiber, potassium and a small amount of vitamin E to the diet. But don't leave out the scallions. Green onions eaten with the tops on contain twice the calcium and iron content, triple the vitamin C and 50 times the vitamin A of mature onions.

Supplies: LONGEVITY BENEFITS *2, 3, 4, 5, 7, 8.*

40-plus frying pan salad

1 tablespoon sweet butter or homemade butter (page 103)

5 cups coarse outer lettuce leaves, cut in strips

2 teaspoons finely chopped mint or 1 teaspoon dried

Pepper and Life Extension Salt (page 106) to taste

¼ cup wheat germ or bran

• Melt butter in a heavy frying pan. Add lettuce and use a wooden spoon to keep it turning until all the leaves are limp and buttery. season with "salt," pepper and mint, sprinkle with germ or bran. Eat warm.

Serves 2.

Uses: Serve with toast and *Stay Young Egg Salad* (recipe below) for a "minimal-calorie" breakfast. Leftovers make a tasty fridge-raider's snack.

Variations: Substitute 1 to 2 cups dark greens (turnip greens, collard or kale) or use 1 cup soaked, drained seaweed in place of lettuce for more time-fighting nutrients. Use corn germ or oat bran in place of wheat.

Stay Young "Egg" Salad: Fork-mash ½ cup mashed tofu, 2 stalks minced celery, ½ cup minced onion, 1 sodium-free chopped pickle, ¼ cup "lite" mayonnaise (50% fewer calories). Spoon into a margarine tub. Add a fork for impulse eating. 10 calories a fork or spoonful.

Stay Young Note: If you're losing weight the Scarsdale way, don't expect to do it at Pritikin prices. The Scarsdale Diet will cost you because that 12-ounce steak on Monday cannot be substituted for the 8 ounces of chicken on Tuesday. The other top contenders aren't any cheaper. If you're looking for a low-cost loser. Here's the diets America's post-30's use most, and how they rate—

Diet	Approximate Cost per Portion (1984 prices)
Scarsdale Medical 14-day Diet	4.77
Dr. Atkins Diet Revolution	4.54
Weight Watchers	1.22
Woman's Doctor's Diet for Women	1.43
Pritikin Longevity Diet	1.84

Supplies: LONGEVITY BENEFITS *1, 2, 3, 4, 7, 8.*

Beta-carotene baked endive

1 pound endive

2 tablespoons butter

⅓ cup water

¼ teaspoon salt substitute

1 tablespoon fresh lemon juice

1½ tablespoons olive oil

Pinch of minced shallots, carrots or green onions

• Place endive in a shallow casserole or baking dish coated with butter. Add water, salt substitute and lemon juice. Dot with butter or olive oil (both supply carotene), cover tightly. Simmer over low heat 15 minutes.

• Uncover and simmer 10 minutes more until lettuce is tender. Spoon olive oil over braised leaves and broil briefly until golden brown. Sprinkle with shallots, carrots or onions, and serve.

Uses: Serve as a light lunch, a super salad dish or a hot "breakfast salad." Also good cold.

Variations: For more beta-carotene, garnish with slices of ripe papaya, cantaloupe or add *Vitamin A Chips* (page 117).

Stay Young Note: Three not-so-healthy foods that are "fair" sources of beta-carotene, according to the National Cancer Institute, are butter, margarine and regular ice cream. Endive is one of the eight foods that get a good-as-carrots rating for carotene.

Supplies: LONGEVITY BENEFITS *2, 3, 4, 7, 8.*

"Stinking rose" soup

24 cloves fresh garlic

3 tablespoons olive oil

2½ quarts vegetable or sea vegetable stock; vegetable cooking water, or reconstituted low-sodium broth or cubes, or miso soup powder

6 lettuce leaves any type, torn

Pepper and/or kelp powder to taste

• Peel garlic (smash with the flat of a large cleaver and the skin will slip off).

• Spoon olive oil into a deep pot or soup kettle. Add crushed garlic and stir over gentle heat, so the garlic will soften without burning (about 5 minutes). Cooking reduces garlic's bite and aroma.

• Add stock and seasonings and bring to a boil. Simmer, uncovered, about 20 minutes. Strain, mashing garlic down to force it through the strainer.

Makes 5–6 servings.

Variations: To turn this recipe into a chicken-colored broth for non-meat-eaters—toss a handful of washed marigold petals into soup 10 minutes before serving or add 1 teaspoon of turmeric or curry powder. Leftovers may be frozen.

Stay Young Note: Without garlic we'd have no pyramids—the colossal wonders of the ages were built by slaves fed with great quantities of garlic. Greek physicians used garlic in their prescriptions and garlic was even rationed to the soldiers of the mighty Rome armies as well as to their slaves and laborers. Among its countless dietary and medicinal virtues, garlic stimulates the appetite, lowers the cholesterol, has a carminative action which means it prevents stomach gas or flatulence. It combats some types of intestinal bacteria and it's nutritious—5.3% protein, 29% carbohydrate (fiber), 1.4 mg. iron in each 4 oz. It's high in potassium, sulphur and cancer-blocking antioxidant selenium, too.

Supplies: LONGEVITY BENEFITS *1, 3, 4, 5, 8.*

Watercress buttermilk soup

2 bunches fresh watercress (about 1 pound)

2 tablespoons unsalted butter

1 cup finely chopped onions

1 teaspoon finely minced garlic

2 cups potatoes cut into 1½ cubes

6 cups vegetable broth

Salt or substitute to taste (optional)

1½ cups buttermilk

Set aside ½ cup of cress leaves to use as garnish.

• Heat butter in a large saucepan, add the onions and garlic. Cook briefly, stirring, until the mixture is wilted. Add potatoes and stir to blend. Add broth and season. Bring to a boil, add watercress sprigs. Simmer about 15 minutes until potatoes are tender.

• Meanwhile, bring about 2 cups of water to a boil and add previously set aside watercress leaves. Simmer 10 seconds, drain and plunge leaves into ice water. Drain once more. Set aside.

• Pour watercress mixture into container of processor or blender and puree. Return soup to pan and heat thoroughly. Stir in remaining cress leaves.

8 or more servings.

Uses/Variations: Chill leftovers for a super-slurper fridge snack.

Stay Young Note: This creamy-no-cream soup is consistent with dietary recommendations made by the American Institute for Cancer

Research, the American Heart Association and the American Health Foundation. A one-and-one-half cup serving has only 150 calories, it's low in saturated fat and cholesterol and it provides the following proportions of the U.S. Recommended Dietary Allowances: protein, 20%; calcium, 25% and vitamin A, 80%.

Supplies: LONGEVITY BENEFITS *3, 4, 5, 7.*

Creamless crucifer soup

4 tablespoons unsalted butter or homemade butter (page 103)

1 medium onion, chopped

1 clove garlic, minced

10 ounces Brussels sprouts,[21] trimmed, sliced lengthwise

1 small fennel bulb,[21] trimmed, chopped

1 teaspoon anise seed, crushed (optional)

2 tablespoons uncooked brown rice

3 cups broth

4 to 6 slices toasted whole-wheat French bread (optional)

4 to 6 teaspoons wheat germ, bran or calcium sprinkles (page 118)

• In a large saucepan over medium-low heat, melt butter and sauté onion till golden. Add garlic and cook 4–5 minutes. Add Brussels sprouts, fennel, anise, rice. Cook, covered, 15 minutes.
• Add broth. Heat to a boil, reduce heat. Simmer, covered, for 30 minutes. Add pepper to taste.
• Place half the sprout-fennel mixture in the container of a food processor or blender; puree until smooth. Transfer to a large bowl. Repeat with the remaining sprout-fennel mixture. Heat through before serving. Or, preheat broiling unit. Ladle soup into individual heat-proof serving bowls. Float a piece of toast atop each serving and sprinkle with wheat germ, bran or *Calcium Sprinkles*. Heat under the broiler until golden.

Serves 4–6.

Uses: Add crackers for a fast, high-fiber lunch. Tote in a thermos with whole-grain breadsticks for a eat-at-your-desk meal.

Variations: Use leeks in place of fennel; substitute cubes of raw, green cabbage for Brussels sprouts.

Stay Young Note: If it grows underground, it probably supplies the cancer-blocking substance called crucifers, says the National Academy of Sciences. All root vegetables from fennel to meat-and-potato "veggies" like carrots are reliable sources of time-fighting crucifers.

Supplies: LONGEVITY BENEFITS *1, 2, 4, 6, 7, 8.*

---

[21]Crucifer source.

Basic soup stock and broth

3 large carrots, diced

5 stalks celery, diced

1 large Spanish onion, quartered

1 large rutabaga, sliced

3 parsnips, sliced

1 bunch fresh turnip greens

1 bunch fresh dill or basil

2 gallons water or 1 gallon water plus 1 gallon Calcium Cup (page 118)

• Combine all the ingredients in a large kettle. Bring to a boil. Simmer, covered, 1 hour. Strain, discarding vegetables, and set aside till cool. Refrigerate.

Makes 1 gallon, enough for 8 servings.

Uses: May be frozen in ice cube trays for a low-cal broth or a base for gravies and sauces for a simple cup-of-soup lunch with crackers or with pureed cooked potato or cauliflower for low-calorie creamed soup.

Variations: Use white turnips in place of rutabaga; substitute broccoli for carrots; use water chestnuts or jicama in place of celery.

Stay Young Notes: The richer your diet is in cabbage and herbs, the poorer a cancer risk you become. According to the National Academy of Sciences, the cabbage patch vegetables used above are top sources of the natural inhibiting substance beta-carotene. They also provide vitamin C, an antioxidant vitamin which blocks the formation of tumors and lowers the risk of cancers of the stomach and esophagus after 30.

Supplies: LONGEVITY BENEFITS 2, 3, 4, 5, 7, 8.

MAIN DISHES

True blue greens (citrus and sea vegetable salad)

Salad:

       3–4 citrus fruits (oranges, grapefruit, ugli, etc.), peeled and chopped

       1 cup dried dulse, rinsed and drained (other sea vegetables may be substituted) (see Variations)

       1½ cups light or dark salad greens

       Rings of raw purple onion

Dressing:

       ⅓ cup safflower oil

       2 tablespoons olive oil

2 tablespoons herb vinegar

1–2 tablespoons lemon juice

½ teaspoon each dried oregano and cumin or cayenne powder

¼ teaspoon kelp powder

• Toss fruits and dulse with dressing and marinate for 15 minutes or longer. Arrange on top of salad greens. Add onion rings. *Optional:* Sprinkle with *Calcium Sprinkles* (page 118), bran or wheat germ.

Uses: With soup, a good cold-grain lunch. Or serve with broiled tofu for supper. Or keep a bowl for help-yourself-fiber-rich-fridge snacking.

Variations: Use fresh kale, grape or comfrey leaves; or a wild green such as plantain or lambs'-quarters; or a different sea vegetable such as nori, kombu or hizicki in place of dulse.

Stay Young Note: One gram of calcium a day is good protection against post-30's hypertension, say Johns Hopkins University Hospital researchers. One cup of sea vegetables or kale provides as much calcium as a glass of milk.

Supplies: LONGEVITY BENEFITS *1, 2, 3, 4, 5, 6, 7, 8.*

Longevity loaf #1

2 cups garbanzo (chick pea) beans, cooked

2 cups lentil sprouts, chopped

2 cups alfalfa sprouts, chopped

2 cups shredded carrots, chopped

½ cup finely chopped celery

½ cup finely chopped onion

½ cup chopped parsley

Juice of 1 lemon

1 or more cloves of crushed garlic, minced

1 tablespoon soy sauce plus 1 tablespoon marjoram

½ teaspoon celery seed, crushed

½ teaspoon kelp or Life Extension Salt (page 106)

1 ripe avocado, peeled and seeded.

• Run garbanzos and lentils through a processor or blender with the lemon juice and soy sauce. Mix all ingredients well. Form into a loaf and chill. Garnish with alfalfa sprouts, fresh parsley and raw vegetable curls.

Uses: Serve as a cold or room temperature meatloaf with Beta-Carotene sweetener or *Soy Sauce* (page 101) for summer lunches/brunches/dinner.

Variations: Use as a pâté, cracker spread or stuff into celery/tomato shells or pita pocket bread.

Stay Young Note: "Bean (sprouted or otherwise)," says Dr. Hans Fisher, chairman of the Department of Nutrition at Rutgers University, "offer top quality nutrition. They are 21% protein, 77% carbohydrate and provide 14 to 18 percent of your protein requirement—to build and repair aging tissues."

Supplies: LONGEVITY BENEFITS *1, 2, 5, 6, 8.*

Longevity loaf #2 (a meatless meatloaf)

⅔ cup brown rice, raw (see cooking note) or ⅔ cup cooked, crumbled tempeh

1½ cups water

⅓ cup sprouted lentils, soy or mung beans, or coarsely chopped wheat

1 small onion, chopped fine

1 small carrot, grated

1 garlic clove, crushed and minced

1 tablespoon parsley, minced

1 tablespoon soy oil or olive oil

1 teaspoon soy sauce (regular or low-sodium)

Season with:

1 teaspoon cumin, ground, plus ½ teaspoon rosemary, ground or crushed

⅛ teaspoon powdered cloves

- Preheat oven to 325°.
- Oven-toast the rice to improve the finished flavor.
- If rice is used—bring water to a boil and stir in rice. Simmer covered for 45 minutes until all the water is absorbed, then cool. Add rice (or tempeh) to remaining ingredients and mix well.
- Press the mixture into 2 small greased loaf pans or 1 large one. Bake for 30–40 minutes until just slightly moist inside. Remove and cool on a cake rack. Slice and serve with *Shake-and-Bake Vegetable Gravy* (page 100) or *Soy Sauce* (page 101).

Uses: Good as a meatloaf or a meatloaf sandwich substitute. May be sliced and frozen for fast-from-the-freezer lunches and dinners.

Variations: If you garden, don't let those greens go to waste. Carrot tops or horseradish greens can be used in place of parsley.

Stay Young Note: There are 120 mg. of vitamin E in half a cup of soy oil (half cup of wheat germ has only 27 mg.).

Supplies: LONGEVITY BENEFITS *2, 5, 8.*

Tempeh rice

½ pound fresh raw tempeh

¼ cup soy oil

¾ cup scallion, minced

⅓ cup green pepper, minced

¼ cup celery, minced

1 tablespoon whole-grain flour

1½ teaspoons garlic, minced

2 teaspoons miso or soy sauce

2 tablespoons red wine

2 tablespoons water

½ teaspoon red or black pepper

1½ cups brown rice, cooked, or ¾ cup each cooked millet and cooked
    cracked wheat (bulgur)

Garnish—mixed sprouts

• Put tempeh through the coarse blade of a food grinder.
• In a large skillet, sauté tempeh in oil over moderately high heat,
stirring for 1 to 2 minutes, or until brown.
• Stir in scallion, green pepper, celery, flour and garlic, and sauté the
mixture for 5 minutes, or until the vegetables soften.
• Add miso paste or soy sauce mixed with red wine, water and pepper.
Sauté, stirring for 3 minutes. Stir in cooked brown rice or millet or cooked
cracked wheat (bulgur). Transfer the mixture to a heated serving bowl.
Sprinkle with fresh mixed sprouts.

Uses: Serve with any Life-Extending salad and *One-Ingredient Bread*
(page 79) for a complete lunch or supper. Save leftovers for a cold brunch or
midnight munching.

Variations: Now that you've tried tempeh, here are a few more ways
to serve it:

• Cut baked or steamed tempeh into "croutons" to make the in-
complete protein of a cold salad supper complete. Add "croutons" to hot
soups and casseroles.
• Crumble tempeh and use as a natural "hamburger helper." Use
filling for tomatoes, cabbage, crepes, green peppers or taco shells.
• Use cooked, crumbled tempeh in place of meat in "Sloppy Joes,"
stirfries, curries, etc.
• For a "time-released" protein-energy diet snack, combine cooked
tempeh and "lite" mayonnaise and spread on whole-grain wafers.

Supplies: LONGEVITY BENEFITS *5, 6, 8.*

No-yolk soufflé

⅔ cup freshly grated Parmesan

3 tablespoons unsalted butter

¼ cup all-purpose flour

1 cup skim or lowfat milk

Nutmeg and freshly ground black pepper to taste

¼ teaspoon hot chili powder, or to taste

4 large egg whites

¼ teaspoon cream of tartar

4 ounces regular or lowfat Swiss cheese, corasely grated (about 1½ cups)

- Preheat oven to 375°.
- Grease a 1-quart soufflé dish and fit it with a 3-inch-high band of foil, doubled and greased, to form a collar that extends 2 inches above rim of dish. Sprinkle dish and collar with 2 tablespoons Parmesan cheese.
- In a small, heavy saucepan, melt butter over moderately low heat, stir in flour with a whisk and cook the "roux" for 3 minutes, stirring. Gradually add milk and keep whisking. Bring mixture to a boil, still stirring. Reduce heat, simmer 2 minutes, add nutmeg, chili powder and black pepper. Remove pan from heat, stir in ½ cup Parmesan cheese and transfer sauce to a large bowl.
- In a separate bowl, beat egg whites until they are frothy, add cream of tartar and continue beating whites until they hold stiff peaks.
- Stir one-fourth of the whites into sauce. Fold in remaining whites and Swiss cheese. Spoon mixture into prepared soufflé dish, and sprinkle soufflé with remaining Parmesan.
- Bake soufflé 30 to 35 minutes, or until it is puffed and golden. Serve immediately.

4 servings.

Stay Young Note: You would have to eat more than a dozen oysters or two small lobsters to match the cholesterol in one egg (250 milligrams).

Almost-eggless buckwheat casserole

4 cups water

2 cups uncooked whole-grain such as buckwheat or bulgur

2 tablespoons oil

1½ cups skim or lowfat milk

5 tablespoons sugar or 2 tablespoons honey

¼ teaspoon ground cinnamon

1 teaspoon vanilla extract

½ teaspoon grated lemon rind

1 teaspoon lemon juice

2 egg whites

2 whole eggs

½ cup raisins

2 tablespoons coconut flakes (optional)

Cinnamon for garnish (optional)

• Preheat oven to 325°.

• In medium-sized saucepan, bring water to a boil, stir in grain, reduce heat, cover pan and simmer until water is absorbed. Transfer to large bowl and stir in oil.

• In medium bowl, beat together milk, sugar or honey, ¼ teaspoon cinnamon, vanilla, lemon rind, lemon juice, egg whites and whole eggs. Add this to grain, stirring ingredients to combine well.

• Stir in raisins, and transfer mixture to a greased 3-quart baking dish. Sprinkle with coconut and additional cinnamon, if desired.

• Bake about 45 minutes until set. Serve warm at room temperature.

12–16 servings.

Stay Young Note: An egg supplies 13 vitamins and four minerals, including vitamins A, B-6, B-12 and D, riboflavin, folic acid, pantothenic acid, calcium and zinc (all of which are found primarily in the yolk). But the quantities are on the small side. The only vitamin that eggs supply in significant amounts is vitamin B-12. Also, yolks are often touted as rich in iron, but their iron is tightly bound to a substance called phosvitin, which prevents your body from readily absorbing it.

Supplies: LONGEVITY BENEFITS *1, 2, 4, 6, 7*

Red-pepper pancakes

2 large red peppers

1 ear of corn

1 shallot, finely chopped (or green onion)

3 tablespoons olive oil

Black pepper to taste

1 cup yogurt

1½ whole-grain pastry flour plus 1 tablespoon brewer's yeast

1 tablespoon baking powder

1 teaspoon Life Extension Salt

1 cup skim milk

3 eggs, separated

Oil for greasing skillet

2 oz. crumbled tempeh or tofu

2 oz. chives

1 oz. fresh coriander (cilantro), dill or parsley

• Grill the peppers briefly over an open flame or under the broiler. Peel and remove the seeds. Chop 1 pepper into a very small dice. Cut the second peper in half and slice half into thin strips. Mince the other half until it's nearly mashed. Set aside.

Sauce

• Remove the kernels from the ear of corn. Sauté kernels, dice pepper and pepper strips and shallot in olive oil for 2 minutes. Season with pepper and add yogurt. Simmer for 15 minutes over medium-low heat.

Pancakes

• Sift flour, baking powder and "salt" into a bowl. Beat egg whites until soft peaks form. Fold them into the egg-yolk mixture, then fold this mixture into the reserved minced peppers mixture.

• Grease a griddle or skillet with oil. Cook 3-inch pancakes over medium-high heat. Keep them warm while you finish batter.

• Serve pancakes with warm pepper-and-corn sauce on top and garnish with chives and fresh coriander, dill or parsley.

Serves 8.

Uses: A meatless main dish for lunch, brunch or dinner.

Variations: And for added life-extension benefits, make "**sourdough**" red-pepper pancakes: Use 1 cup prepared commercial sourdough start and omit ½ cup of flour and ½ cup of liquid, and the baking powder in recipe above.

Stay Young Note: What are the four sources of calcium in the fancy flapjacks above? Corn, yogurt, milk and tofu/tempeh. Like to add three or four more? Garnish with slices of one of the new exotic high-calcium fruits in your supermarket fresh produce department: cherimoya; Asian pear and soursop (all tropical fruits) or try one of the new acid oranges: Lavender Gem and Blood Oranges.

Supplies: LONGEVITY BENEFITS *1, 2, 5, 6, 7, 8.*

SIDE DISHES/SNACKS

It isn't always meals that age you faster—it's snacks. Watch those I'm-50-I've-paid-my-dues-and-I-deserve-a-break-today chips and dips. Here's what a few of the *usual* can do: 1 ounce tortilla chips: 150 calories; 1 ounce potato chips: 160 calories; 1 English muffin with butter: 252 calories; 1 cup grape juice: 160 calories; 1 cup cottage cheese: 239 calories; 2 ounces Cheddar cheese or 10 cheese straws: 250 calories; 1 ounce salted roasted almonds: 178 calories; 2 tablespoons peanut butter: 200 calories; ½ cup granola: 260 calories; 8 ounces whole-milk fruit yogurt: 260 calories.

Solution? Switch to homemade.

Roots of health apple sauce

4 Golden Delicious apples (about 2 pounds)

¼ cup natural sweetener (dry)

¼ cup water

3 tablespoons horseradish root (see note), freshly grated, or 1 tablespoon prepared horseradish.

• Peel the apples and quarter. Cut away and discard the stems and cores.

• Cut each quarter crosswise into thin slices to make five to six cups. Put slices in a saucepan and add sweetener and water. Bring to a boil and simmer 10 minutes or until the apple slices are tender.

• Pour cooked apples and juices into the container of a food processor or electric blender and puree. When cool, add in horseradish.

2 servings.

Uses: As a side dish for meat or meatless entree; a non-sweet dessert, or snack, a chip dip.

Variations: Use over cold desserts such as pudding instead of whipped cream.

Stay Young Note: Horseradish is a root to root for if you're avoiding the rocking chair. It supplies Vitamin C—a long-life nutrient that's destroyed by aspirin, caffeine, alcohol and stress. It tastes best and nourishes most when recently harvested and freshly grated. Horseradish should be kept in vinegar, if not used immediately to prevent discoloration—or after grating it, place it in a container of water and refrigerate or wrap it in a wet towel and keep in a plastic bag. You can also plant leftover root outside until further use.

Supplies: LONGEVITY BENEFITS *1, 2, 3, 4, 5.*

Life-extension rice

2½ cups Basic vegetable stock (see page 87)

3–4 sliced green onions (include green part)

1 cup brown rice

¼ cup sweet corn kernels, fresh or frozen

¼ cup instant non-fat dry milk (increases protein and adds crunch)

1 cup chopped tomato

¼ cup fresh basil, chopped

¼ cup chopped water chestnuts

• Combine stock and onion in large saucepan and bring to a boil. Stir in rice. Reduce heat, cover and simmer for 30 minutes. Add corn, dry milk, tomato, basil and chestnuts. Simmer about 10 minutes, or until grain is tender.

Serves 4.

Uses: As a hot side dish or a cold chip-attack substitute.

Variations: Substitute buckwheat or converted white rice in place of brown; use chopped nuts in place of water chestnuts; use parsley in place of basil.

Stay Young Note: One-quarter cup of brown rice supplies 88 milligrams of magnesium which makes it a healthier magnesium booster than peanut butter, apricots or Swiss chard. A diet deficient in magnesium contributes to the risk of kidney stone formation, according to the *Journal for Vitamins and Nutritional Research*, 44 (3) 74.

Supplies: LONGEVITY BENEFITS *3, 6, 8.*

Red hots (radish stirfry)

1 pound (about 3 cups) unblemished red radishes, trimmed of stems
  and leaves[22]

2 tablespoons corn oil

1 clove garlic, crushed, minced

Kelp or Homemade Salt (page 106)

Freshly ground pepper to taste

½ cup finely chopped green onions or leeks

• Cut radishes into thin slices.

• Heat oil in a skillet. Add sliced radishes, garlic, kelp or homemade salt. Cook about 3 minutes, tossing and stirring so radishes cook evenly.

• Add green onions or leeks. Grind on pepper. Continue cooking, stirring and tossing for an additional 2 minutes until radishes are *al dente.*

Serves 4.

Uses: Serve hot as a salad, main dish or side dish. Keep in the fridge as a "free food" diet snack.

Variations: Use white or black radishes or the Oriental radish Daikon which is high in vitamin C. Or mix any two radish types.

Stay Young Note: Make that wok or skillet stainless steel, add a little lemon juice and you'll add life-lengthening chromium (a trace mineral),

---

[22]Save the nutrient-rich leaves for your next salad.

too. The body can turn chromium into GTF (the glucose tolerance factor), also found in brewer's yeast, which helps prevent maturity-onset diabetes.
Supplies: LONGEVITY BENEFITS *1, 2, 3, 4, 5, 8.*

Nucleic acid chip-dip chips (a no-sodium chip with the no-fat dip built in)

• Slice one large, fresh zucchini squash in very thin slices. Spread with a thick layer of thick, homemade or store-bought yogurt. Sprinkle generously with brewer's or nutritional yeast powder or flakes and/or *Life-Extension Salt* (page 106).

• Dehydrate for approximately 15 hours or until dry at 135–140° in a home dehydrator (see *Mail Order Sources*), under a hot sun, or in a low (120–150°) oven (keep door ajar) overnight. When chips are crisp and dry, store in a jar on a dry shelf.

Uses: A chip, a cracker substitute or serve crumbled in soups and salads.

Variations: For a "Nacho" flavor: mix yeast with paprika and salt-free curry or cumin powder to taste. And for a saltier flavor, sprinkle with powdered kelp; use yellow summer squash in place of green zucchini. Or try chayote, a mild and crunchy "new age" squash in produce departments of better supermarkets.

Stay Young Note: Brewer's yeast supplies twice as much time-fighting nucleic acids as sardines, the second best source.

Supplies: LONGEVITY BENEFITS *2, 3, 4, 5, 6.*

Oven onions

10 medium onions (about 5 pounds)

10 tablespoons olive oil

1 teaspoon chopped garlic

½ teaspoon red-pepper flakes

2 tablespoons chopped parsley

Pinch freshly ground black pepper

1 teaspoon vinegar

1 teaspoon Life-Extension Salt (page 106)

• Cut onions into ⅝-inch-thick slices, leaving skin on. Put onions on an oiled heavy baking sheet, brush very lightly with olive oil, bake at 300° for one hour. Turn slices with a spatula, and continue baking for 30 minutes. Onion should be caramelized, not burned.

• Use a spatula and transfer slices to a wide, shallow serving dish. Remove skin, any "dried out" rings and mix remaining oil with garlic, red-pepper flakes, parsley, 4 tablespoons water, pepper, vinegar and "salt." Spoon over onions. Serve at room temperature.

8 to 10 servings.

Uses: Serve as a good, fast-food snack, a salad aside, a sandwich topping.

Variations: Substitute a nut oil for olive oil; use lemon juice in place of vinegar.

Stay Young Note: Peeling onions is nothing to cry about if you eliminate the propanethial-s-oxide they contain. P-S-O is a volatile gas that is released when an onion is cut or bruised. To prevent tearing, pre-chill the onion and slice them under running water or wear goggles.

BEVERAGES

After 30, most of what we drink is on the health-seekers endangered species list—alcohol, caffeinated coffee, soft drinks, cocoa, hot chocolate.

Here are some healthier ways to keep refreshed without raising your blood fats, blood pressure, lowering your blood sugar levels or adding stress to your life.

Live-longer ginseng milkshake

1 packet (or 2 teaspoons) granulated ginseng

Hot water

1 small banana, chopped

1 cup skim milk

2 ounces unsweetened fruit juice

2 coops sugar-free ice cream or yogurt

• In a large glass, dissolve the ginseng in a small amount of hot water. In a blender, mix banana, milk, fruit juice. Add ginseng and ice cream or yogurt.

Variation: Use ½ cup strawberries instead of banana.

Stay Young Note: Two to three glasses of milk per day offers some protection from colon rectal cancers by raising your calcium and vitamin D levels, says Dr. Cedric Garland and his colleagues at the University of California at San Diego. (But to avoid raising cholesterol levels, use non-fat.)

Supplies: LONGEVITY BENEFITS *1, 2, 4, 5, 6, 7.*

Atomic tea

2 cups cold brewed ginseng tea (see Variation)

3 cups fresh melon, cut in chunks, fresh (see directions below) for melon juice

2 tablespoons fresh mint leaves

• Blend mint and tea. To make melon juice, puree chunks of melon in the blender.

• Blend with the tea and milk. Serve over ice. To boost the energy effect, add 1 teaspoon bee pollen granules for each 1 cup serving.

Uses: As a Gatorade substitute, as a "get-going" cola substitute or a low-calorie liquid snack.

Variations: Instead of just ginseng, use an herbal blend such as ginseng/gotu kola/ginseng-comfrey or ginseng-peppermint (using either one small, peeled ripe cantaloupe or a combination of 2 melons such as casaba and honeydew or Persian and musk).

Stay Young Note: When you *do* decide to drink non-herb tea, make a low-caffeine choice. Here's the punch three favorites pack: China teas (Earl Grey; black currant; China oolong): 10% to 20% of the caffeine of coffee; Breakfast and Indian teas (English and Irish breakfast and Assam): 30% to 40% of the caffeine of coffee; Green teas (green gunpowder and jasmine are your best choices with only 2% to 7% of coffee's caffeine).

Supplies: LONGEVITY BENEFITS *1, 2, 4, 5, 6.*

Health cola (sugar-free, caffeine-free)

8 tablespoons black cherry concentrate,[23] undiluted

7 cups salt-free club soda or sparkling water

2 teaspoons lemon juice

Ice cubes or crushed ice

Orange, lemon or kiwi fruit slices

Honey (optional)

• In a pitcher, mix fruit concentrate, lemon juice and soda. Add ice, garnish with fruit slices. Taste. Sweeten if desired.

Makes 8 servings (about 45 calories each).

Uses: Serve as a cola or iced tea alternative.

Variations: Add 1 teaspoon angostura bitters; substitute lime juice for lemon.

Or substitute undiluted grape juice concentrate.

Supplies: LONGEVITY BENEFITS *3, 4, 5, 6.*

Longevity lemon water

1 quart sparkling mineral water

---

[23]Natural fruit concentrates are carried by most health food stores.

Juice of ½ a lemon

1 tablespoon freshly cracked peppercorns

• Pour mineral water into a clean, empty wine bottle and add freshly squeezed lemon and peppercorns. Chill, serve in wine goblets.

4 servings.

Uses: A saccharin-free diet drink, a no-alcohol cocktail.

Variations: Use lime or grapefruit, kiwi or mango juice in place of lemon; use seltzer or salt-free club soda in place of sparkling water.

Stay Young Note: Never give the lemon the raspberry. Did you know the American lemon tastes acidic because they are picked when green and ripened off the tree, not on? Or that heavier lemons taste better and juicier? Or that lemon juice makes an effective antacid substitute?

Supplies: LONGEVITY BENEFITS 3, 4, 6.

SAUCES, SPREADS, DIPS

Two fried hamburgers supply 40 grams of saturated fat and almost 400 mg. of cholesterol—more than twice the dose per meal—that the American Health Association calls healthy.

The sauces you add and dips and spreads you use may be just as bad. There are almost 7 grams of fat in popular brands of canned beef gravy; for example, 17 in chicken gravy—and hollandaise sauce prepared from a mix has more fat than spareribs. And America's favorite herb-tomato sauce has as much fat as a small fast-food ice cream cone.

Storebought may be *out* if you love buttery sauces, good gravies and spreads. But here's what you can use in its place to lower fat and cholesterol in your diet.

Sauce and Dips

One-calorie vegetable dip

1 whole artichoke

1 cup fresh green beans or raw asparagus tips and stalks

1 cup water or vegetable broth

Juice of ½ a lemon

1 shallot, minced

1 or more garlic cloves, crushed

1 teaspoon dried marjoram plus 1 teaspoon basil

• Combine all ingredients in a small, deep saucepot and cook 20 minutes until tender.

• Remove artichoke and cool. Spoon pan juices into a dip dish and serve with choke. One calorie a tablespoon.

Uses: Hot as an all-in-one vegetable and dip dish or side dish or snack, or use the broth with beans or asparagus as appetite-stopper broth.

Variations: Artichokes are lean, green longevity food. Only 30 calories each with twice the potassium and iron of most diet-lite green veggies. Asparagus and stringbeans are a close second. Substitute either.

Stay Young Note: The greener the spear, the more tender the asparagus texture will be and the higher yield per pound. And don't pay top dollar. Three pounds of costly nearly-all-white asparagus spears yields less than 12 ounces of good-looking asparagus. You get the same 12 ounces of edible asparagus from only 1 pound of all-green spears, says the USDA. And a 10-second test for freshness? Sniff the tips. If they smell, buy a choke instead.

Supplies: LONGEVITY BENEFITS *1, 3, 5.*

Shake-and-bake vegetable gravy

3 cups skim milk or lowfat milk

8 tablespoons cooked, pureed vegetables: i.e., onions, potatoes, corn, carrots, parsnips or a combination (avoid vegetables with strong flavors and odors such as cabbage and Brussels sprouts and turnips)

Cayenne, nutmeg and poultry seasoning or Life-Extension Salt (page 106) to taste

• Combine ingredients in a screw lid jar and shake vigorously to blend or puree until smooth in the blender. Add to saucepan; heat, stirring with a whisk until puree is thick and smooth.

5 servings.

Uses: A substitute for the usual high-fat/high-calorie, flour-and-egg-thickened sauces/gravies. Spoon over steamed vegetables, rice or cooked pasta.

Variations: Use as a cold dip for homemade chips and vegetable sticks.

Stay Young Note: Mushroom gravy in a can has 10 grams of fat. The kind you reconstitute has 4. And both have more sodium than 4 ounces of pork sausage (1 gram). The above is a more fruitful way to sauce with no fat at all.

Supplies: LONGEVITY BENEFITS *1, 2, 3, 4.*

Sauces

Soy sauce, sauce #1

1½ cups soy milk or lowfat milk

2 teaspoons miso (soybean paste)

2 tablespoons mushrooms, chopped

1 tablespoon carrot, grated

1 tablespoon chives or rosemary crushed

• Combine first two ingredients in blender. Puree. Add to small saucepan with remaining ingredients. Bring to a boil, reduce heat, simmer and stir using a wire whisk for 5 minutes.

Soy sauce, sauce #2

3 tablespoons unsalted butter or butter substitute

¼ cup onions, chopped

1 cup tofu, crumbled

1 teaspoon garlic, crushed

¼ cup white wine

6 oz. soy milk or skim milk

Pinch of nutmeg

1 teaspoon regular or low-sodium soy sauce

1 teaspoon dried rosemary or 1 tablespoon fresh chopped

• Melt butter and sauté onions until soft. Add crumbled tofu garlic and blend well. Whisk in the wine and milk and bring to a boil. Season to taste. Puree sauce until smooth. Reheat, stirring. Reduce heat and simmer 5 minutes.

Uses: Serve with any vegetarian entree such as tofu or tempeh, or mixed vegetable dish, spoon over open-faced sandwiches.

Variations: Use crumbled pre-cooked tempeh in place of tofu in Sauce #2; substitute brewer's yeast concentrate for miso (look for Marmite brand in supermarkets) in Sauce #1.

Stay Young Note: Getting rosemary into your diet often? The most useful of all mediaeval garden herbs, it has added sass to salads since mediaeval times. Its natural oils, suggesting the aroma of pine woods, nutmeg and heliotrope with a hint of ginger, are used as an extract, tea, tincture or seasoning. It is one of history's garden patch cures for dropsy, a weak circulation, insomnia, heartache and headache. And in sickness and in health, nothing's tastier. Outside the salad bowl? Combine chilled rosemary tea and lemonade and spike with orange peel.

Supplies: LONGEVITY BENEFITS *2, 4, 6, 7.*

"Avocado" sauce (guacamole substitute)

2 cups cooked asparagus tips

Juice of 1 lemon

2 teaspoons fresh chopped tarragon or ½ teaspoon dry

1 tablespoon olive oil or Longevity butter (page 103)

2 tablespoons yogurt or soft-type tofu

Red pepper (cayenne) to taste

• Puree asparagus tips. Beat in lemon juice, tarragon, and yogurt; mix to a creamy paste. Correct seasoning; chill. Thin (if needed) with skim milk.

2 cups sauce.

Uses: Chip and cracker dip, a cold summer soup, a low-cal/low-sodium cup-of-soup for breakfast.

Stay Young Note: Guacamole can use up your fat allowance for the day. Two of those buttery alligator pears provide 40 grams of fat—the maximum the government recommends. This healthier version is practically fat-free.

Supplies: LONGEVITY BENEFITS *1, 3, 4, 5.*

"Cheese" sauce

1 lb. tofu

2 tablespoons sesame butter

¼ cup plain yogurt

1 teaspoon nutritional yeast

2 tablespoons soy sauce

1 tablespoon safflower oil

1 teaspoon lemon juice

• Combine all ingredients and blend until smooth. Spoon into covered refrigerator dish.

• *To make sauce*: Puree 2 tablespoons of base with 1 or more cups skim milk, vegetable broth or vegetable juice. Transfer to saucepan and heat, stirring until sauce is thick.

Uses: Spoon over toasted muffins; use in casserole dishes calling for "melted cheese."

Variations: To make Cheese Spread Substitute, just prepare the base and chill in a covered refrigerator container. Use as a bread spread or spread on top of pizzas and other baked dishes in place of sliced cheese.

Stay Young Note: The buttery cheese sauce above made without cheese or butter has only 5 grams of fat a serving. Keep that rarebit and fondue on the menu.

Supplies: LONGEVITY BENEFITS *3, 4, 5, 6.*

Eggless eggs benedict sauce

½ cup nutritional or brewer's yeast (flakes or powder)

1 teaspoon lecithin granules (for smoother consistency)

¼ cup whole-grain flour

⅓ cup soy, corn or olive oil

2–3 tablespoons soy sauce

Water, vegetable broth or Stock (recipe page 87) as needed

¼ teaspoon fresh ground pepper or cayenne

• Put yeast, lecithin granules and flour in a heavy skillet and toast over low surface heat stirring with a whisk. Add oil gradually and continue to stir until sauce bubbles and browns. Add water and stir until sauce is the correct consistency. Season to taste with soy sauce and pepper.

6 servings.

Uses: If the first meal of the day has come and gone, use this sauce on steamed root vegetables or sea vegetables or to spoon over open-face sandwiches, or thicken with 2 tablespoons of whipped cottage cheese or tofu and use as a dip.

Variation: For a darker gravy-like sauce, blend in 1 teaspoon miso.

Stay Young Note: One serving of eggs benedict sauce has more fat than two fast-food strawberry sundaes, and twice the amount of cholesterol the American Heart Association considers safe. The recipe above sauces those eggs without the extra eggs, cheese and cream.

Supplies: LONGEVITY BENEFITS *1, 3, 5, 6.*

Sauces/Spreads

Longevity butter

Note: Butter, margarine and buttery juices are loaded with cholesterol and calories. But even fats from vegetables such as avocados and palm plants, have been found to cause cancer, especially of the colon and bowel, says the Center for Science in the Public Interest. Polyunsaturated oil can be hazardous to your health, too. Sound extreme? National Cancer Institute studies indicate that laboratory animals fed liquid vegetable oils in their diets in place of solid fats suffered a greater rate of cancer than those fed saturated animal fats. What to do? Give up bought butter and make your own safer "clarified butter" for cooking called "Ghee". Used in non-western countries for centuries, this "better butter" below doesn't bubble or smoke, contains no additives and won't go bad (bad butter can be a source of carcinogenic free radicals). Homemade is sweeter, more delicately flavored and gives you more vitamin A than other table fats.

Directions

• Place 1 pound of good quality (Grade AA) whipped, sweet (salt-free) butter in a heavy saucepan. Melt on burner or in a hot oven. Stir and bring to a slow boil.

• When a layer of foam appears on the surface, lower heat and continue to cook down undisturbed for 60 minutes in a low oven. Butter will separate, and under the layer of solid white surface foam there will be an amber-colored butter. At the bottom of the saucepan, some sediment collects because the water has evaporated and the protein solids have separated.

• Without shaking the pan, use a fine mesh wire skimmer and skim off as much as you can. Strain the clean liquid through several thicknesses of cheesecloth to remove remaining foam.

• Ladle into a glass jar or crock with a tight-fitting lid. Refrigerate or freeze. At low temperatures, longevity butter becomes solid. One pound of bought butter yields 1½ cups melted homemade.

Uses: A melted butter substitute, a vegetable dip.

Variations: Make *Longevity Butter Plus*: Add 1 tablespoon of *Garlic or Onion Puree* (page 105) or 1 teaspoon fresh or dried salad herbs to each 1 cup of butter; insted of 1 pound of grade AA butter, use 1 pound soybean margarine from the health food store (free of saturated fats).

Stay Young Note: Another plus—this butter may be heated to a higher temperature than most oils or fats without smoking because the water, which normally bubbles at 212°F, has been removed. Protein solids generally reach a smoking point at about 250°F in fats and oils, and these are gone, too.

Supplies: LONGEVITY BENEFITS *1, 6*.

Spreads

Beta-carotene cream cheese (dairyless cracker spread)

1 cup raw sunflower seeds

1¼ cups water

Cayenne (red pepper), garlic, onion or shallots, oregano parsley, savory or thyme, basil, dried or fresh

Optional: carrot juice or turmeric

• Puree seeds, herbs and water in blender. Ferment the mixture in an open or cloth-covered jar (a Mason or mayonnaise jar is fine) at room temperature for 24 hours. When air bubbles develop, do a taste test. Flavor should be sour, tart, lemon-like. Pour out any excess water on top. You now have a dairy-free "nut yogurt."

• Place cheese in a triple layer of cheesecloth, tie up and suspend over the sink to drip-dry at room temperature (70–75 degrees) overnight.

• Conventional cream cheese has 10 grams of saturated fat an ounce. This alternative spread is fat-free. For a more carotene color, add a squirt of carrot juice or a pinch of turmeric, or crushed marigold petals if you're a windowsill gardener.

Uses: A bread and cracker spread, a dip, a stuffing for sandwiches, celery and cucumber, artichokes.

Variations: For a sharper cheese, add a pinch more flaked or granulated garlic or cayenne after draining. For spicy flavor, add extra oregano, dill, thyme or basil; spread and dry as directed.

Stay Young Note: What do high-fat cheese, heavy aspirin intake and cancer have in common? The first two contribute to the third by depleting the body store of beta-carotene, the vitamin A precursor named after carrots. To protect yourself, keep plenty of vitamin A-precursor-rich foods on your menus. The one that's highest in carotene and lowest in calories? Parsley.

Supplies: LONGEVITY BENEFITS *2, 3, 4, 6.*

SEASONINGS AND SPREADS

Garlic or onion purée

8 garlic bulbs or 2 large bulb onions, peeled and cut in chunks

1 tablespoon olive oil or safflower oil

• Put garlic bulbs in steamer basket. Place over boiling water in saucepan. Cover; steam 30 minutes. Separate and peel cloves. Mash the cloves. Combine crushed garlic and oil. Refrigerate. Substitute bulb onions, cut in chunks. Puree in blender or food processor.

Garlic or onion butter

• Beat together ½ cup softened sweet butter (or use *Longevity Butter*, page 103, and 1 teaspoon *Garlic or Onion Puree*, page 105). Use as a topping for hot cooked vegetables; use as a chip dip.

Makes ½ cup.

Garlic/onion oil

• Place 1 large peeled and crushed head of garlic or 1 small coarsely grated bulb onion in a jar with olive oil to cover. Keep on a warm shelf three days. Shake twice daily. Strain through a fine sieve and use flavored oil for cooking or as a vegetable mixture to fight flatulence and the common cold.

Garlic/onion grass (chives)

• Plant individual unpeeled cloves or shallots (pointed ends up) in clay pots in shallow, rich but sandy soil 6 inches apart. Cover loosely with plastic wrap.
• Water daily. When green shoots appear, harvest by clipping with scissors. (Flavor is gentle, so is the odor.)

Use on salads, in yogurts, soups, over baked potatoes, or add to butter for garlic-chive-butter spread.
Supplies: LONGEVITY BENEFITS *1, 3, 4.*

Life-extension salt I (low sodium seasoning)

1 cup sesame seeds

1 tablespoon powdered kelp

• Wash seeds. Drain. Scatter over bottom of a thin-bottomed skillet and toast over a medium-hot burner until seeds snap, crack and brown. Pour into blender jar, add the kelp and grind to a powder. Store in a spice jar.

Uses: Salt substitute and MSG-free flavor enhancer.
Variations: Substitute another powdered sea vegetable such as dulse or spirulina for kelp or use powdered vitamin C.
Stay Young Note: A 3-ounce serving of salty-kelp provides over 1 gram of osteoporosis-preventing calcium, the mineral regular table salt depletes. Sesames are the best seed source of calcium.
Supplies: LONGEVITY BENEFITS *1, 4, 5, 7.*

Life-extension salt II

½ tablespoon each cayenne pepper and ground cloves

1 tablespoon each cinnamon, ginger, nutmeg, cumin, coriander and
   dry mustard

2 tablespoons each curry powder, sweet paprika and ground white
   pepper

3 tablespoons each granulated onion, granulated garlic

Pinch of natural dry sugar (optional)

• Combine all ingredients and keep in a tightly covered container in refrigerator or freezer. Use as is or mix with regular salt or commercial salt substitute.

Uses: As a salt, seasoning or a raw vegetable/hard-boiled egg "dip."

Variations: Make a *Life-Extension Bread Spread*: Blend 1 teaspoon *Life-Extension Salt* into a cup of soft butter.

Stay Young Note: Three good liquid salt substitutes? Angostura bitters, low-sodium soy sauce and Tabasco sauce.

Supplies: LONGEVITY BENEFITS *1, 5.*

DESSERTS/DESSERT TOPPINGS/SWEETENERS

Loaded for bear claws and doughnuts? Indulge. Sinkers can be healthy if you bake them, don't fry them yourself.

So can candy if you leave the sugar, chocolate and fat behind. *Any* dessert you love as much as life itself can improve your health and lengthen your life—in fact, here's how:

Time-fighting ice milk (calorie-trimmed and sweetener-free)

1 6-oz. can frozen, unsweetened orange juice concentrate

1 6-oz. can frozen, unsweetened pineapple juice concentrate

3½ cups cold water

1 teaspoon pure vanilla

1 cup nonfat dry milk, yogurt powder or buttermilk powder

Optional: 1 teaspoon powdered vitamin C or calcium ascorbate powder or acerola powder (natural vitamin C from acerola berries)

Wheat germ or bee pollen, 1 to 3 tablespoons

• Beat all ingredients except wheat germ to blend thoroughly.

• Pour into ice cube trays sprinkled with pollen or wheat germ; freeze one to two hours. When half-frozen, transfer to a chilled mixing bowl; beat at low speed until softened, then on high speed 3 to 5 minutes until mix is just creamy. Fold in pollen or wheat germ and optional ingredients if used.

• Spoon back into trays, freezer containers or popsicle molds. Cover with foil and freeze until ready to eat.

10 fat-free servings.

Uses: A 75-calorie-a-dish dessert. Healthy enough for a hot, summer breakfast.

Variations: Three healthier-than-chocolate-ice cream sprinkles? Maple syrup granules, carob chips, toasted Grape-Nuts.

Stay Young Note: A lickety-split for longevity? Your best bet is store-

bought Glacé. It's 50% fruit, 98 calories a half cup, less sodium and fat than any other frozen dessert and it's milk- and saccharin-free.
Supplies: LONGEVITY BENEFITS *2, 3, 4, 7.*

Anti-aging oatmeal cookies

1 cup almond butter (or tahini or peanut butter)

½ cup maple syrup or honey

¼ cup unrefined sunflower or safflower oil

1 tablespoon vanilla

⅓ cup water

1 cup rolled oats

1 cup quinoa flour[24]

½ cup toasted almonds, chopped

9 whole almonds

Pinch of salt or Life-Extension Salt (page 108)

• Preheat oven to 375°F. In a mixing bowl, blend almond butter, sweetener, oil, vanilla and water. Sift together flours and salt, add chopped almonds and combine with wet mixture.
• Using hands, form dough into small balls and place on an oiled cookie sheet. Press each cookie gently with the tines of a fork. Cut whole almonds in half and press one piece, cut side up, into each cookie. Bake for 12 to 15 minutes or just until golden.

Makes 24 cookies.
Uses: Serve as a dessert, a high-protein calcium-booster snack.
Variations: In place of quinoa, use another super flour such as amaranth or triticale. Second best choice—whole wheat or whole rye.
Stay Young Note: Quinoa flour, which is ground from a millet and sesame-like seed that is 3,000 years old, has 141 mg. of age-proofing calcium per 4 ounces compared to wheat's 36 and corn's 6. It also has more fiber and protein.
Supplies: LONGEVITY BENEFITS *6, 7, 8.*

40-plus pudding

4 cups unsweetened fruit juice

1 bar agar-agar (sea vegetable gelatin)

1 tablespoon tahini (sesame butter)

---

[24]Available from Sproutletter Publications (see *Sources*) or Walnut Acres (see *Sources*).

• Combine the ingredients. Bring to a boil. Turn off the heat. Let cool. Pudding will solidify at room temperature. Spoon custard through a blender. Spoon into popsicle molds or dixie cups with sucker sticks.

Uses: Serve as a dessert or breakfast pudding or make *50-Plus Popsicles*: Pour pudding before it sets into dixie cups and freeze till almost solid. Insert sucker sticks.

Variations: Substitute peanut butter or another nut butter (sunflower seed, almond, cashew) for tahini.

Stay Young Note: Are you out of agar-agar? Substitute plain gelatin, but put this jello-of-the-sea on your shopping list. Best reason besides taste and convenience? It puts more than twice the calcium into your diet than cow's milk and without adding saturated fat, says the Japanese Nutritionists Association.

Supplies: LONGEVITY BENEFITS *3, 6, 7, 8.*

Forty-plus tomato sauce/tomato ice

2 pounds tomatoes

1 tablespoon honey

Juice of ½ a lemon

6–8 basil leaves

• Blanch the tomatoes in boiling water for 1 minute. Remove from boiling water and rinse with cool water to stop cooking. Peel, quarter and seed the tomatoes.

• Place tomatoes in a blender with honey, lemon juice and basil, and puree. This mixture should be pleasantly tart. Add more lemon juice or honey as necessary. Divide mixture between two ice-cube trays and freeze.

• To serve, chill sherbert glasses or glass bowls in freezer. Thaw cubes for 10 to 15 minutes. Place cubes in a blender or food processor a few at a time. Puree until the ice is small-grained and slightly slushy. Scoop into chilled serving dishes and garnish each portion with a sprig of basil.

Makes 3 cups.

Variations: Make *Long-Life Fruit Ice*: Use 2 pounds of peeled, seedless oranges (better than everyday O.J.'s? Try acid-free lavender oranges or the grapefruit substitute, ugli fruit) in place of tomatoes; substitute fresh, flat-leaved parsley or dill weed for basil.

Stay Young Note: The Italians call an ice like this a *granite* and serve it as either a tart, light dessert or a healthy palate-refresher between courses. But if you've been good and deserve a "bad food" break today, have a Fudgesicle instead. Only 90 calories and it satisfies 16 percent of your RDA for calcium.

Supplies: LONGEVITY BENEFITS *3, 4.*

Pineapple "sauerkraut"

· 2 cups natural sugar (date sugar or maple syrup granules, et al.)

6 cups water

1 fresh pineapple in chunks or slices or 2 cups drained canned pineapple

1½ teaspoons whole anise, crushed

1 teaspoon cloves, crushed

3-inch stick cinnamon

Plain yogurt

• In a large glass container or crock, combine all ingredients and stir to combine well.

• Cover loosely. Ferment for 3 days, stirring well once a day.

• Taste, strain (reserve the juices for a pancake/French toast dribble), chill. Stir in plain yogurt before serving.

Makes 7 cups.

Uses: As a dessert, snack or a meat substitute side dish.

Variations: Papaya and/or mango may be substituted for pineapple.

Stay Young Note: This is a sugar-free version of "Tezween," a Lebanese longevity drink rich in the health-boosting natural digestive enzyme—bromelain.

Supplies: LONGEVITY BENEFITS *4, 6, 7.*

Seeds of health "salami"

½ cup pure honey

¾ cup ground poppy seeds

½ cup sesame seeds

1 cup ground walnuts

¼ teaspoon ground clove

¼ teaspoon ground cinnamon

Coating: bee pollen, 6 tablespoons (optional)

• Bring honey to a boil, preferably in top of double boiler.

• Add remaining ingredients and blend well. Let cool.

• Turn mixture out on a dried pastry board (even better, a cold marble slab). Roll in pollen granules (if used) and wrap in waxed paper. Chill thoroughly. Cut into 32 bite-sized slices.

Uses: A rich after-dinner or between-meal sweet; an after-exercise energizer.

Variations: Substitute chopped sprouts, reduce honey to ½ cup and add ¼ cup *Whole-Wheat Sweetener* (page 116)

Stay Young Note: A five-ingredient, no-additive candy like the above which you can make is hard to find. The eight easy-to-find candies below have as many calories and lots of unhealthy fats:

Product	Serving Size	Calories
Cadbury Almond or Hazelnut bar	2 oz.	310
Butterfinger	2 oz.	290
Charleston Chew	1.8 oz.	220
Hershey's Milk Chocolate	1.45 oz.	220
Kit Kat	1.5 oz.	210
Natural Licorice bar	1.3 oz.	135
Jelly Belly Jelly beans	25	100
Pearson's Coffee Nips	1 piece	30

Supplies: LONGEVITY BENEFITS *1, 4, 6.*

Healthy whole bran halva

1 cup lightly roasted, shelled sunflower seeds

4 tablespoons bran or germ (wheat, oat or corn)

½ cup pure honey

• Grind sunflower seeds in a nut mill or blender until fine. Mix in bran, place in skillet over low heat[25] for 5 minutes, stirring constantly to prevent burning. Add honey, cook 5 minutes until moisture in honey evaporates. Spread the mixture in a buttered dish and let it cool until hard. Cut into 12 bite-sized squares.

Uses: A snack, a cookie substitute or serve with fruit for dessert.

Variations: To make a higher calcium halva, use cashews or peanuts in place of sunflower seeds and add *calcium sprinkles* (page 118) or 2 tablespoons of milk or yogurt powder.

Stay Young Note: This bit-of-honey Italian torrone substitute is sugar-free—and even better, the bran in it is a heart-health-booster.

Supplies: LONGEVITY BENEFITS *5, 6, 7, 8.*

Anti-aging apples (apple-miso dessert)

5 apples, peeled and quartered lengthwise

1 cup water

1 tablespoon miso paste

½ cup raisins

---

[25]According to University of Kentucky studies, as little as 4 ounces of bran a day added to an otherwise typical American diet for 10 days can cut cholesterol levels in the blood by as much as 25%. The major ingredient is the fiber *beta glucans*.

1 tablespoon lemon juice

2 tablespoons honey

2 tablespoons sesame or peanut butter

¼ teaspoon cinnamon or other dried herb

½ bar of agar (4 to 5 grams), soaked 5 minutes, squeezed dry and chopped

• Combine apples and water in a saucepan, bring to a boil and simmer, covered, for 10 minutes.

• Using a fork, remove apples and transfer to a baking pan or mold. Add miso and the next five ingredients to the apple cooking liquid, mixing well.

• Add agar, bring to a boil and simmer for 4–5 minutes, until agar has dissolved.

• Pour liquid into mold and cool to room temperature. Cover, refrigerate until firm. Serve with yogurt or *Whipped Tofu Topping* (page 115).

5 to 6 servings.

Uses: As a cold fruit dessert or a hot, instead-of-cereal alternative.

Variations: Substitute five large, firm pears or two papayas for apples; use 1 tablespoon gelatin in place of agar.

Stay Young Note: In your 30's, start a low-fat, high-fiber diet to protect yourself against heart disease, cancer and other ailments. The 30's mark the beginning of your body's decline, says Harvard University Medical School's Dr. John Rowe. Apples, agar and raisins are three top sources of fiber.

Supplies: LONGEVITY BENEFITS 2, 3, 6, 7, 8.

Life-extension vinegar-and-date pie

Filling:

½ cup sweet butter, softened or homemade substitute

2 tablespoons unbleached or whole-wheat pastry flour

1¼ cups date "sugar" (dehydrated dates), firmly packed, or 1 cup natural cane sugar (see Sources)

2 eggs

½ cup apple juice

¼ cup apple cider vinegar

¼ cup crushed walnuts or pecans, use for extra crunch (optional)

1 scoop soy ice cream or Tofu Whipped Cream (see below)

Crust: Use a prepared pie crush shell (or use any cracker recipe in this book). Press crust gently into 9-inch pie pan. Set aside.

- Preheat the oven to 375°F.
- In a medium-size bowl, cream together the butter, flour and sweeteners until light.
- Add eggs, beating well after each addition.
- Stir in apple juice and vinegar and blend well. Pour filling into crust, sprinkle with chopped nuts.
- Bake for 50 to 60 minutes until the filling is set (a knife inserted into the center will come out clean). Top with scoop of an ice cream substitute or *Tofu Whipped Cream* (place 1 cake of tofu in blender with 1 tablespoon undiluted frozen fruit concentrate or 1 tablespoon honey; puree till light).

12 slices.

Uses: A meal's end dessert or a tea-time sweet.

Variations: Substitute wheat sprouts or granola for nuts; divide dough and filling in half and bake as two turnovers instead of one pie.

Stay Young Note: The original version of this recipe dates from a bygone era. Vinegar and lots of "bad" brown sugar added tang to the gooey, super-sweet filling. In this version, you use dried dates or calcium-rich cane sugar to make it sweet but healthier.

Supplies: LONGEVITY BENEFITS *6, 7, 9.*

Vitamin C croissants

¼ cup unsalted butter or Homemade Butter (page 103)

1 tablespoon fresh-grated lemon peel

½ teaspoon vitamin C powder (optional)

4 whole-wheat croissants, split lengthwise

1 cup orange juice, reconstituted double-strength

¼ cup natural sugar (powdered maple syrup, malt granules, etc.)

3 tablespoons extract (orange, vanilla, almond, etc.)

- Mix butter and peel in small bowl. Spread 1 teaspoon mixture on 1 cut side of each croissant; close croissants. Bake in pre-heated 325° oven for 10 minutes.
- Meanwhile, in small saucepan boil remaining butter, orange juice and sweetener 5 minutes until syrupy. Place croissants in a skillet. Pour on syrup, keep hot. Heat in a low oven until warm.

Serves 4.

Uses: With skim milk, 120-calorie breakfast or brunch with tea, a 350-calorie dessert.

Variations: For *Super-C Croissants*: Add ½ teaspoon C powder to the syrup before spooning on; substitute papaya or cranberry juice for O.J. For crunch plus C? Add crushed walnuts to the syrup.

Stay Young Note: Good sources of C besides citrus? Try papaya (twice the C of grapefruit), green peppers, guava (more C than melon and berries) and common herb teas such as sage, mint, parsley and rosemary.
Supplies: LONGEVITY BENEFITS *4, 8,*.

Vitamin P parfaits (3 life extension fruit cocktails)

#1—Pineapple sauced with strawberry puree
Cut off the top and bottom of one ripe pineapple. Slice off the brown skin, removing any eyes. Cut the pineapple into wedges, working around the core. Place in a champagne glass and top each wedge with 2 table-spoons pureed, thawed frozen (or fresh) strawberries and a sprinkling of natural (brown not red) pistachio nuts or toasted bran flakes.
#2—Pink grapefruit with blueberry sauce
Peel and section a large pink grapefruit with a sharp knife. Place in parfait glasses. Puree 1 cup of thawed frozen blueberries with 1 tablespoon raisins. Spoon puree over grapefruit. Garnish with thinny-thin slices of lemon or lime peel.
#3—Oranges with ginger-yogurt sauce
Peel and section one large seedless orange. Set aside. Mix ½ cup plain lowfat yogurt with reserved juice and ½ teaspoon freshly grated ginger. Spoon sauce evenly into 2 parfait glasses, arrange orange sections on top and garnish with finely grated lime or orange peel. Sprinkle with toasted poppy or sesame seeds or bee pollen.
Uses: Dessert, diet snack, a healthy breakfast in a hurry.
Variations: Use any of the above as fruit dips, cone-stuffers, blintz or crepe fillings.
Stay Young Note: How does a juicy-fruit dessert lengthen your life? By reducing your calorie intake. Each has 100 calories or less per serving and boosts your day's intake of vitamin P, also known as the bioflavonoid factor, that is part of the vitamin C complex. The desserts above provide anti-cancer fruit fiber, too, in the form of pectin.
Supplies: LONGEVITY BENEFITS *1, 3, 4, 6, 8.*

50-plus creme fraiche

1 cup crumbled, drained tofu

2 tablespoons plain, thick yogurt

• Combine tofu and yogurt in a small saucepan. Mix thoroughly using a wire whisk. Heat over very low heat until just barely lukewarm (about 85 degrees on a cooking thermometer).
• Pour into a scalded jar; cover and let stand at room temperature until thick throughout on the bottom when you test with a chopstick or knife blade. (Don't overferment.) Thickening may take 8 to 24 hours depending on room temperature. A temperature of 80° is perfect. Cream

should thicken in 12 hours at this temperature (and it thickens a bit more once refrigerated).

• When the cream tastes done, stir thoroughly and refrigerate 8 hours before serving. Chilled, it lasts up to 14 days.

Makes 1 cup of topping.

Uses: Because it's fermented and lower in fat, this is a healthier version of the famous French dessert. Similar to sour cream but less acid (10 calories a tablespoon vs. 60 calories for creme fraiche). Use as a sour cream and whipped cream substitute, a fruit topping for pie and berries, fruit cocktails and puddings, or use as a dip.

Variations: Stir in dried fruit and serve for a fruit cocktail-with-topping-built-in dessert.

Stay Young Note: Watch those other storebought creams you buy, too. Here are the calories and cholesterol they supply:

	Calories (per 4 oz.)	Cholesterol (mg.)
Plain yogurt	74	15
Cream cheese	420	75
Sour cream	225	75
Whipped cream	416	163

Supplies: LONGEVITY BENEFITS *3, 5, 7, 8.*

Tofu whipped cream

1 cup soft tofu, crumbled

3 tablespoons dry curd cheese, farmer's cheese or uncreamed cottage cheese

2 tablespoons mild honey or rice syrup

½ teaspoon vanilla extract

¼ cup water, as needed.

• Combine all ingredients in blender and process till smooth and creamy.

Uses: A whipped cream substitute for topping puddings, pancakes and fruit cocktails, or eat "as is" as an ice cream alternative.

Variations: For tangerine-colored whipped cream, use *Beta-Carotene Sweetener* (page 116) in place of honey; for *Black 'n Blue Whipped Cream,* add 2 tablespoons pureed fresh or drained-frozen berries, cherries or grapes.

Stay Young Note: Storebought tofu-based frozen desserts contain as many as 300 to 500 calories a cup. Have a cup of the above instead, top with *Calcium Sprinkles* (page 118) and you're 200 calories or less.

Supplies: LONGEVITY BENEFITS *3, 5, 7.*

Beta-carotene liquid sweetener

8 oz. freshly squeezed or canned carrot juice

2 tablespoons undiluted orange juice concentrate

• Combine ingredients. Refrigerate.

Uses/Variations: Use as a honey or corn syrup substitute, as a topping for sundaes, yogurt, fruit cocktail, pancakes; as a substitute for both the milk and sugar on hot and cold cereals.

Stay Young Note: Eight ounces of super-sweet carrot juice provides up to 50,000 units of anti-cancer, better-night-sight beta-carotene. Take 1 tablespoon daily for a beta-carotene-vitamin boost.

Supplies: LONGEVITY BENEFITS 2, 3, 4, 7.

Wholewheat sweetener

(*Note*: Toasting improves fiber and increases the natural sweetness in whole grains.)

2 cups rolled oats

1 cup sugar and salt-free wheat flakes

Water or herb tea (about ¼ cup)

Cinnamon or pumpkin pie spice to taste

Wheat germ or bee pollen

• Preheat oven to 325°F. Dampen cereal flakes with water or tea. Pat dry.

• Spread flakes in a thin layer in a shallow baking pan or on a lightly greased cookie sheet. Place in the oven to toast about 20 to 30 minutes. Stir twice to prevent overbrowning. Blend in cinnamon or pumpkin pie spice and wheat germ or pollen if used.

• Cool mixture. Grind in blender until powdery. Store in a tight container.

About 3 cups.

Uses: Use as you would brown sugar or maple sugar. (But use more. This is only a fifth as sweet.)

Variations: To increase sweetness and add antioxidants vitamins A and C, put in dried fruit that has beeen dried twice: Spread 1 cup any dried fruit, finely chopped, on a cookie sheet. Dehydrate overnight in a 120–150° oven. Process next day to a powder using food processor or food grinder and add to powdered cereal; substitute corn or rye flakes for wheat.

Stay Young Note: Did you know that every year 12 to 16 tons of teeth are extracted in the United States alone? And that repairs on the teeth that are left in place account for $2 billion in dental costs? The reason? Sugar. According to the Center for Science in the Public Interest, America's intake has risen 224% since 1900. When you need a pick-me-up, pick a healthier sweet food with a high glycemic rating (that means it boosts your energy but doesn't rot your teeth). A glycemic rating refers to a food's ability to raise your energy by increasing the sugar levels in your bloodstream. The five that do what sugar does—but not as fast and without ruining your teeth—are carrots, parsnips, plain cornflakes, white potatoes and shredded wheat.

Supplies: LONGEVITY BENEFITS *1, 5, 6, 8.*

Vitamin A chips

1 small fresh pumpkin

Pinch red peper (cayenne)

2 tablespoons honey

Wheat germ or dry milk powder

• Cut pumpkin in half. Remove strings and seeds from each half. Bake in preheated 300° oven until tender. Scrape meat from the shell and put in blender with pinch of red pepper and honey. Blend until smooth. If very watery, thicken with wheat germ or dry milk powder.

• Spoon puree on two cookie sheets covered with cooking parchment or plastic wrap. Dry in a low oven overnight or longer. Better yet, dry in your food dehydrator following manufacturer's directions. When pumpkin is very dry and chewy, it's done. Break into chips and store in glass jars.

Uses: As a french fry alternative, or vitamin supplement snack.

Variations: Substitute any other vitamin A-rich vegetable such as winter squash, carrots, chayote squash or vitamin A fruit such as cherries or apricots.

Stay Young Note: Dried foods are health foods. One-half cup of banana chips from the supermarket provide five times as much vitamin A as one fresh banana and seven times as much iron. Storebought alternative: banana chips, sweet potato chips, carrot chips or sea vegetable snack crackers are all fun food sources of life-lengthening vitamin A.

Supplies: LONGEVITY BENEFITS *2, 3, 4, 6, 8.*

Homemade vitamin D

• Beat 2 egg yolks or 2 whole eggs until light and pour onto a greased earthenware plate. Dry until brittle under a hot sun, in a warm oven or a dehydrator, then grind or pound to a powder. Add toasted wheat germ.

Uses: 1 tablespoon a day sprinkled on toast, cereal, fruit or vegetables.

Variations: Spread in a thin layer on a greased earthenware platter or flexible cookie sheet with sides. Dry in a warm oven. Break into 24 bite-sized pieces and grind in a meat mill or electric grinder.

Stay Young Note: Cholesterol worry-wart? Don't be. Did you know that your dehydrator makes egg yolks a good source of healthy blood fat-lowering lignin, gum and hemicellulose—three of the five top food fibers?

Storebought Alternatives: 2 fresh egg yolks or 1 tablespoon fish liver oil; or order yolk and whole egg powder (it keeps without refrigeration) from Now Foods (see *Sources*).

Supplies: LONGEVITY BENEFITS *4, 5, 7.*

Calcium cup (an old-fashioned way to take your calcium on the half shell)

• Place one fresh raw egg (shell intact) in a glass of good-quality white vinegar. After three days, the shell will dissolve. Discard the egg, add the vinegar solution to 2 quarts of plain water or mineral water. Sweeten with honey and lemon juice to taste. Liquefy in blender.

6 to 8 servings.

Uses: A calcium supplement to sip or cook with. Use to thin cream soups and gravies and boost their calcium content.

Variations: Substitute a fruit-flavored vinegar such as raspberry or tarragon for white vinegar.

Stay Young Note: An egg shell contains about 2 grams of calcium. Plain water won't coax it out, you need acid. If you're out of vinegar, a soup made with an acid fruit or vegetable such as tomatoes or lemons will do. The amount of calcium which is dissolved into the vinegar depends on the level of the acid in the food and the length of time the shell soaks.

Storebought Equivalent: If you'd rather have somebody else do the processing, egg shell calcium powder is available at health food stores (see *Sources*).

Supplies: LONGEVITY BENEFITS *1, 5, 7.*

Calcium sprinkles

• Toasted sesame seed
• Kelp powder
• Parsley flakes
• Dried vegetable flakes and dehydrated soup vegetables
• Horseradish
• Pistachio nuts
• Calcium carbonate or calcium lactate powder
• Red pepper flakes or powder
• Sunflower seeds
• Wheat bran or oat bran
• Maple syrup granules

- Wheat germ
- Peanuts or almonds, flaked or crushed
- Chopped raisins
- Soy granules
- Dried lemon or orange peel
- Skim or whole milk powder
- Parmesan cheese
- Buttermilk, yogurt or sour cream powder (Saco is one brand super-markets sell)
- Powdered whey
- Agar-agar flakes or powder
- Oyster shell powder or eggshell powder
- Barley leaf juice powder (Green Magma)
- Dried fish flakes

• Use the above alone or in combinations with or without salt *Life-Extension Salt* (page 106) in your shaker. A few grains of rice added to the shaker prevent clumping.

• One healthy shake provides 20 to 50 mg. of calcium. Use liberally on everything from salad and soups to nuts, snacks and desserts.

Stay Young Note: Americans consume more ice cream than any dessert-happy country in the world. Eighty-six percent of our freezers stock it. Does it belong in your longevity freezer? You bet. Ice cream is a first-rate source of *calcium*, something 50 percent of all older women need more of, says Louis Avioli, M.D., director of the Division of Bone and Mineral Metabolism at Washington Unviersity in St. Louis and at the Jewish Hospital of St. Louis. Calcium prevents osteoporosis, the shrinking bone disease common in women after age 40. To get two-thirds of the 800 to 1,500 mg. of calcium a day you need—have a double dip of vanilla ice cream and sprinkle with calcium-rich wheat germ.

Supplies: LONGEVITY BENEFITS *1, 2, 4, 5, 7, 8.*

3

Staying Young Nutrients and Supplements

STAYING YOUNG NUTRIENTS

Every organ and tissue in your body requires not one but dozens of nutrients to maintain high-level wellness as you age. Vitamin E, for example, increases post-40 male potency, improves the circulation, oxygen capacity and stamina, helps your body heal its wounds and builds your anticancer immunity, but not unless you're getting it in doses of 400 milligrams or more, which few foods provide.

Vitamins' functions overlap—vitamin A, C and the mineral magnesium all help shield you from stress while vitamin thiamine (vitamin B-1) and iron help each other keep your mind sharp. No vitamin, in fact, performs one job and one job alone. Vitamin B and C both prevent fatigue, for example. All nutrients work together for your total long-life good. If they're all present and accounted for, you'll feel good. If you have just one post-30 health problem, you may not. If your memory's failing, you need an additional 100 to 400 milligrams of B-6 plus 5 to 20 milligrams of manganese a day to curb forgetfulness. You can't get that easily from food alone. If your body's low in C, you won't be able to make good use of whatever amount you do have. Result? Anemia and chronic fatigue, says Dr. Lendon Smith. Rx? An extra 100 mg. of B-12 a day—something you'll never get unless you do something nobody does—put organ meats (kidney, sweetbreads, liver, etc.) on your menu daily.

Not that longevity begins with vitamin A and ends with zinc. Iron's a must. Adequate iron levels in the body fight infection, improve mind and

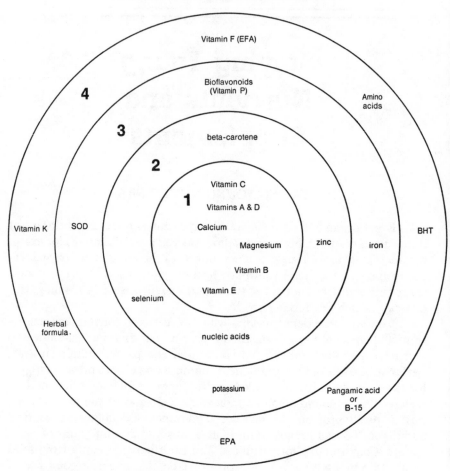

THE STAYING YOUNG NUTRIENT TARGET:
BEST VITAMINS AND MINERALS FOR LIFE EXTENSION

- Circle 1 and 2 — recommended daily supplements.
- Circle 3 — suggested supplements.
- Circle 4 — optional supplements.

Figure 3-1

memory, prevent hair loss and anemia which causes energy losses, even ward off some forms of cancer. Iron absorption is increased by adding vitamin C to meals and cutting down on tea and coffee, which block the body's uptake of iron. Protein's important, too, because it's a source of time-fighting amino acids. And according to Dr. Roy Walford, a shortage of amino acids such as methionine found in aged brains, contributes to premature senility. Amino acids, the building blocks of protein, minimize the effects of oxidation which weakens immunity and DNA repair. Another amino acid youthful people swear by is *cysteine* in 300 mg. tablets. You also get it when you eat eggs, soybean foods and sea vegetables such as kelp.

Ready? Here are 15 nutrients that do the most to help you slow the aging process down to a walk.

15 FOOD SUPPLEMENTS THAT HALT THE AGING PROCESS

- *Vitamin C/Bioflavonoids*
    - Increase Your Lifespan by 12–18 Years
    - Are Your Bad Habits Lowering Your Vitamin C Reserves?
    - The Orange Juice Vitamin That Cleans Your Arteries
    - Vitamin C Fights the Big C
    - Is Your Body Manufacturing the CSA It Needs?
    - How Vitamin C May Save Your Sex Life after 40
    - Boost Your Life-Extending Vitamin C—Take Bioflavonoids, Too
    - Vitamin C-Takers' Tips
    - Top Sources of Vitamin C and Bioflavonoids
- *B Complex*
    - 24 Conditions That Respond to B-Complex
    - B-1: The Anti-Senility Nutrient
    - Are You Low in These Four Easy-to-Get B Vitamins?
    - How One Week of B-Complex Meals and Supplements Can Make You Feel Young Again
    - Take More B If You're Blue
    - Conditions and Situations That Can Make You B-Vitamin Deficient
    - Tips on Boosting Your B-Intake Daily
    - Why the USDA Studies Indicate You Need to Supplement, Too
    - Best Sources of B-Complex

- *Beta-Carotene, Vitamin A and D*
    - Beta Carotene Foods Reduce Cancer by 25% or More
    - What's the Difference Between Animal Vitamin A and Vegetable Vitamin A?
    - Improve Your Youthful Appearance in a Month or Less
    - Determine Your Vitamin A Needs and Don't Forget D
    - How to Get Enough of "Both" A's from Meals and Snacks
    - 10 Ways Vitamin D Helps Slow Aging
    - Top Sources of Vitamin A and Beta-Carotene
    - Top Sorces of Vitamin D
- *Vitamin E*
    - Why You Need More Vitamin E After 40 to Fight These Four Age-Related Ills
    - Six More Reasons You May Need More Vitamin E After 30
    - Four Ways to Reverse Varicose Veins Without Drugs
    - Vitamin E and Fibrocystic Breast Disease
    - The Magic Grain That Adds Vitamin E to All Your Meals
    - Four Environmental Reasons to Boost Your Vitamin E Intake
    - Top Sources of Vitamin E
- *Calcium*
    - High-Calcium Foods Can Increase Your Life by 10 Years
    - What the National Institute on Aging Says About Calcium and Aging
    - Why Women Need More Calcium Than Men
    - Older Men Benefit from Extra Calcium, Too
    - Best Calcium Sources According to the American Heart Association
    - Good Double-Value Calcium Foods
    - Mineral Takers' Tips
    - Top Sources of Calcium
- *Magnesium*
    - Why Low Magnesium Levels Increase the Risk of Heart Disease
    - The Canadian National Research Council Advises More Magnesium for the Active
    - Six Benefits of More Magnesium
    - Seven Magnesium Snacks That Boost Youthful Vigor

- Take the Amount That's Healthiest for You
- Best Sources of Magnesium
- *Zinc, Selenium, BHT, SOD, B-15*
  - Trace Minerals Help You Win the Bad Habit Battle
  - Antioxidants Prevent Post-30 Body Rust
  - Big Magic Comes in Minimum Doses
  - The Miracle of Selenium
  - Too Little Zinc Leads to Rapid Aging
  - Tipoffs You're Suffering Zinc Deficiency
  - What the Metabolic Research Foundation Says About SOD
  - A Good Food Additive That Fights Aging
  - Scientific Studies Say B-15 Improves Your Immunity
  - Why You Need Supplements to Get Antioxidants in Your Diet
  - Top Sources of Antioxidants
- *Herbs*
  - The Secret of the World's Oldest Young People
  - A Good No-Calorie Source of Staying Young Minerals
  - Fight Bad Breath, Arthritis and Osteoporosis with Parsley Tea
  - 10 Benefits of Ginseng
  - Rejuvenate Your Senses with Herbs
  - Herb Tea, the Antacid Alternative
  - Eat the Flowers to Reverse PMS, Poor Sight, Vitamin Deficiencies
  - Top Sources of Herbs

VITAMIN C AND THE BIOFLAVONOIDS

Double your pleasure, improve your periodontal health and lengthen your life. You can do all three with increased vitamin C. According to the Linus Pauling Institute, optimum amounts of vitamin C (up to 10 grams a day) could increase your life expectancy by 12 to 18 years.

Short of longer life, ascorbic acid does plenty over the short haul to keep you healthy. More ascorbic acid strengthens blood cells that fight infection and it combines with iron to make it unavailable to oral bacteria which need iron to cause decay and the gum problems associated with aging that we know as periodontal disease. According to Dr. Millicent Goldschmidt, associate professor at the University of Texas Dental Branch's Dental Science Institute, Houston, Texas, periodontal disease includes gingivitis and pyorrhea which both destroy gum tissue and cause jaw bone deterioration, the country's number-one midlife dental crisis.

The Orange Juice Vitamin That Cleans Your Arteries

Other good reasons to get more than the ultra-conservative 60 mg. the RDA calls for? Today's food supply doesn't provide enough. Hunter-gatherers of the caveman days consumed four times more ascorbic, acid-rich food than modern man, says anthropologists Dr. S. Boyd Eaton and Melvin Konner of Emory University in Atlanta, Georgia. Vitamin C is one of what Washington heart specialist Dr. James Anderson calls, "the 6 artery cleaning factors" that prevent heart disease—the nation's top life-short-ener.

Are Your Bad Habits Lowering Your Vitamin C Reserves?

The pills in your life are another reason for vitamin C deficiencies. (See chart, pages 155-7.) Medications that deplete your body's store of vitamin C include aspirin and its substitutes, cortisone, laxatives and diuretics,[1] hypertension drugs, alcohol and nicotine. Caffeine also reduces vitamin C absorption so drink your morning juice and coffee at least one hour apart to benefit from the C in the juice. The very nature of vitamin C is another reason to take more than 60 mg. a day. Vitamin C is water-soluble—i.e., you urinate and sweat it away. You also lose C when you overcook, soak food too long or expose them to excess light and heat. Potatoes lose 70% of their vitamin C when deep-fried, for example.

Vitamin C Fights the Big C

In healthy enough doses, ascorbic acid remedies and prevents numerous age-related ills. Vitamin C aids in the formation of collagen, the fibrous tissue found throughout the body that maintains capillaries, bones and teeth; it protects other vitamins from destruction, and it improves the body's absorption of iron. Vitamin C is even a painkiller. According to Dr. Ewan Cameron of Scotland who gave large doses of vitamin C to five cancer patients who were also getting drugs, "They stopped asking for morphine, because the vitamin C was controlling their pain. And they had no withdrawal symptoms. Appetites improved and they lived longer than predicted."

Vitamin C can cancer-proof your body as well, by blocking the formation of cancer-causing nitrosamines. And according to Dr. Linus Pauling, "Taking 10 grams a day (10,000 mgs) would insure a 10% decrease in age

---

[1]Vitamin C is a good substitute for a diuretic. At doses above 5 grams, it works as a laxative as well without boosting blood pressure or causing edema, advises the Pauling Institute.

mortality for cancer patients and a 50% decreased incidence of cancer among normal populations." Pauling himself takes 10 grams of vitamin C daily. One payoff—you'll experience new stores of energy as you increase your dosage, says Pauling.

Your heart benefits, too. According to an 11-year study in Norway, the dietary habits of 16,713 people were monitored. During that period, 43% of them died from stroke. And what did the stroke victims leave out of their diet that survivors didn't? Vitamin C-rich fruits and vegetables, say the study's directors, Dr. S. E. Vollsett and Dr. E. Bjelke of the University of Berten in Norway.

Is Your Body Manufacturing the CSA It Needs?

Vitamin C protects your heart as it ages in other ways, says Anthony Verlangieri, Ph.D., associate professor of pharmacology and toxicology at the University of Mississippi, by helping the body manufacture a chemical compound called CSA which acts as a kind of mortar in healthy artery walls. Cholesterol only damages artery walls that lack CSA. "CSA can prevent over 1 million heart attacks a year," says Lester M. Morrison, M.D., former director of the Institute for Arteriosclerosis Research at Loma Linda University School of Medicine in California. And the best way to obtain it is to get more vitamin C to manufacture it. And if you're taking it for your heart, consider timed-release ingestion. Research by Alacer Laboratories in California indicates that vitamin C is lowest in your body at 4 a.m., the time when the most heart attacks occur.

How Vitamin C May Save Your Sex Life After 40

Vitamin C may save your post-40 sex life. Studies by University of Texas medical researchers indicate that the dose that restores failing fertility in less than a month is 1000 mg. of vitamin C a day.

You need all the C you can get if you get sick because your body absorbs less vitamin C when your resistance is low due to interaction of plasma proteins and endotoxins produced by the bacteria. Your body activates a substance that inhibits vitamin C absorption necessary for healing, reveal studies at the Temple University School of Dentistry. That means the amount of vitamin C that meets your needs when you're healthy isn't enough, says Dr. Joseph Alec, professor of pathology.

Boost Your Anti-Aging Vitamin C—Take Bioflavonoids, Too

To get A-1 protection from C, it's best to get the bioflavonoids, too, which constitute the rest of the vitamin C complex. Dr. Albert Szent-Gyorgyi, the scientist credited with discovery of vitamin C found in 1936 that crude preparations of ascorbic acid from citrus fruits were more effective in preventing capillary fragility than the purified vitamin. This so-called "Flavone factor" was first called "Citrin" and was isolated in citrus fruits and in Hungarian red peppers (paprika) in conjunction with ascorbic acid. Some 140 flavone compounds naturally occur in plants.

The bioflavonoids (sometimes called "vitamin P") strengthen the tiny capillaries throughout the body making them less permeable. They also protect against histamine shock in allergy, help prevent stroke and also potentiate the value of vitamin C protecting it against destruction. Bioflavonoids help lower blood pressure by dilating the arterioles in the heart. Taken with vitamin C they help counteract the effects of toxins, and are also helpful in reducing stress.

What's a healthy amount of vitamin C plus bioflavonoids? Up to 15 grams is safe. And one gram a day is a good amount to start with if you're healthy.[2] But that doesn't mean the sky's the limit.

Vitamin C-Takers Tips

Here are the most frequently cited (and most frequently disrupted) side effects of too much vitamin C:

• Formation of calcium-oxalate kidney stones and precipitation of gout. There's a test your doctor can administer to establish whether this is a problem for you.

• Taking high doses of C then stopping them may cause "rebound scurvy" (deficiency), including bleeding gums. So once your body gets comfortable with an amount and you're healthy, it's best to stick with it.

• Interference with anticoagulants. If you're on anticoagulant medication, discuss C supplementation with your doctor. Large doses could interfere with its effectiveness.

• Vitamin C may inhibit detection of hidden blood in the stool and urine. If you're preparing to take such tests, stop your vitamin C supplementation 72 hours beforehand.

• Diarrhea. When you've taken more vitamin C than your body can handle, flatulence and diarrhea may result, but your digestive system gradually adapts so don't worry.

Once you decide on a dose, what form should you take? The best one may be calcium ascorbate or buffered C, advises the *Journal of American Dental Association*. The worst forms are chewables because vitamin C is extremely acid and chewing it will cause erosion of the enamel on your teeth. The time-released kind can be a plus, too. Vitamin C is water-soluble so your body doesn't store what it doesn't use which makes it safe but also makes it mandatory that you replace what you lose.

---

[2]Better than guessing if you're getting enough, buy a vitamin C test kit and check on how much C your body's really absorbing from food supplements (see *Health Gadgets*, page 221).

Top sources of vitamin C and bioflavonoids

- Lemons
- Grapefruit[3]
- Oranges[3]
- Limes[3]
- Kiwi fruit
- Papayas
- Cauliflower
- Kale
- Spinach
- Fennel
- Asparagus
- Zucchini
- Red peppers[3] and paprika
- Buckwheat[3]
- Strawberries
- Guava
- Chili peppers[3]
- Broccoli
- Brussels sprouts
- Parsley
- Cabbage
- Beet greens
- Artichokes
- Radishes
- Sprouts
- Daikon (oriental radish)

Note: An Australian fruit that looks and tastes like English gooseberries, called *Terminalis ferdinandiana* or "manmohpan" may be Mother Nature's top source of C. The fruit is ¾-inch long and less than a ½ inch in diameter, varies in color from light green to yellow and contains a single large pip or seed. Laboratory tests reveal that three samples of the fruit showed vitamin C contents of 3, 150, 2,850 and 2,300 mg. in 100 grams of the fruit (about 3½ ounces). (Oranges have ⅟₅₀ that amount.) This super and high-C fruit can't be grown outside Australia so your next all-natural

---

[3]These are good bioflavonoid foods, too.

bets in the meantime are Acerola cherries (1,000 mg. in 100 g.), rosehips (500 to 6,000 mg. in 100 g.) or one large bell pepper, guava or orange (about 125 mg. each). All are available in single or in combination supplements.

B VITAMINS

24 Conditions That Respond to B-Complex

"All that stands between you and the possibility of developing diseases such as depression, poor hair growth, confusion, memory loss, conjunctivitis, photophobia, skin disorders, heart disease, poor circulation, poor digestion, loss of gastrointestinal musculature, arthritis, poor nail growth, poor coordination, muscle soreness, general aches and pains, insomnia, allergies, hypoglycemia, anemia, neuritis, fatigue, malaise and weakness is less than an ounce worth of a family of chemical substances known as the B-complex vitamins," says Arnold Fox, M.D., internist, cardiologist and assistant professor of medicine at the University of California at Irvine.

B-1: The Anti-Senility Nutrient

The B-complex vitamins are essential to growth reproduction, energy and a healthy immune system. After 30, B-1 vitamin deficiencies can lead to senility. In a second study at Mount Sinai Hospital in Manhattan, rats deprived of thiamine for two weeks demonstrated neurological symptoms after only 10 days. On the fourteenth day, researchers supplemented the rats with thiamine. "Thiamine administration completely reversed the (serotonin-related) changes in the brain within two days, which coincided with the clinical improvement of these animals," they reported.

Are You Low in These Four Easy-to-Get Life-Extending B Vitamins?

According to University of Mexico researchers Drs. Elizabeth Root and John Longenecker, while a deficiency of vitamin B-6 (along with the mineral copper) causes rats to show the same brain cell abnormalities as senile humans, inadequate intake of B-12, folate and riboflavin (B-2) can do the same. Healthy, mature individuals with a low intake of these four easy-to-get vitamins scored significantly lower on mental tests than those with adequate amounts.

Being caught with your B-1 levels (thiamine) down can be bad for other reasons. According to Derrick Lonsdale, M.D., of the Cleveland Clinic Foundation, who studied a group of men and women with depression, insomnia, chest pain, recurrent fever and chronic fatigue, blood tests revealed that each patient was suffering from severe thiamine deficiency brought on by eating large quantities of refined carbohydrates without taking in enough additional B-1 to metabolize (burn up) the junk food calories. The body experiences this kind of imbalance as a thiamine shortage when it is repeated often enough, says Dr. Lonsdale, producing nervous symptoms characteristic of beriberi, the classic thiamine deficiency disease. All patients improved after being put on a daily dose of thiamine.

How One Week of B-Complex Meals and Supplements Can Make You Feel Young Again

Becoming a B-keeper pays off. Symptoms you may have thought you were stuck with for life may vanish in less than a week of B-complex supplementation, supported by B-vitamin-rich meals—hair that's not gray today or tomorrow, for example. According to hair specialist and trichologist Phillip Kingsley, "Laboratory tests have shown that a deficiency of vitamin B causes grayness, and that reintroducing B vitamins (especially inositol) to the diet may restore normal color." How does Kingsley feed his customer's hair back to natural color and health? With large doses of brewer's yeast and defatted dried liver, the two best sources of B-complex.

Take More B If You're Blue

Mid-life blues are another reason to get more B complex, suggests Dr. Humphrey Osmond, a professor of psychiatry at the University of Alabama, whose experience in treating depressed patients with B vitamins has convinced him that they "help you cope better." (A good "beat-the-blues" formula that "beats drugs" couples at least 1 gram of C with at least 1 gram of B-complex a day.)

Conditions and Situations That Can Make You B-Vitamin Deficient

When you're pushing back the sands of time, the B's to be the most concerned with are B-1, B-2, B-3, B-5, B-6 and B-12. The USDA suggests your RDA for these B's at midlife is 5 mg. Researchers, such as Karl Folker of the University of Texas Institute for Bio-Medical Research in Austin, say it's not enough to cover normal need let alone abnormal ones. Dr. Folker uses 300 mg. or more to provide drug-free relief from nighttime muscle spasms, joint stiffness and swollen feet and ankles, even neurological disorders such as carpal tunnel syndrome.

One reason it's safe to take larger amounts of B-complex is that you lose a lot of what you take through elimination and perspiration. Another reason, according to the USDA's Human Nutritional Research Center on Aging, is that as the intestinal system ages, absorptions of nutrients such as folic acid and B-1, B-2 are impaired, so you need to take more to get enough. "Studies show levels are lower than in younger individuals."

Fractions of B-complex, such as B-6, are also lost if you use penicillin, diet drugs, or contraceptives, diuretics, caffeine or alcohol. And what's true of one B vitamin is generally true of the rest. Too much alcohol, too much medication and too little B-1 rich-foods result in a slowdown in calcium absorption, for example, while B-12, the energy-rich red blood B, is destroyed by such diet additives as salt substitutes made from potassium chloride.

Tips on Boosting Your B-Intake Daily

Getting enough B-complex is easy. Even if you hate B-rich liver or are allergic to the yeast or soy that most natural B supplements are made from—there's bound to be a B-complex food and supplement you can live with. A good one to consider: rice bran which might be considered the first natural food supplement. The word "vitamin" was coined by Casimer Funk back in 1911 to describe the concentrate he produced from rice bran that prevented beriberi. Rice bran is sold as a cereal and a powder to add to blender drinks or baked goods in place of flour, and several vitamin companies offer rice-bran-based B-complex.

Why the USDA Studies Indicate You Need to Supplement, Too

But don't count on getting a natural live-longer amount of *any* B-complex vitamin from food alone. To meet the even skimpiest standard set by government sources for B-6, for example, suggests USDA home economist Martha Laurie Orr, you would need to eat more than two cups of filberts, or buckwheat flour, or one whole cup of sunflower seeds, adding diet-busting calories to your diet days.

Take at least one B-complex tablet that provides 100 mg. of each of the B's, or a capsule at breakfast or lunch. And introduce some of the following foods into your meals on a daily basis.

Best sources of B-complex

- Brewer's yeast
- Wheat germ
- Organ meats (liver, kidney, heart, etc.)
- Egg yolk
- Green, leafy vegetables
- Nuts
- Whole-grain bread and cereal
- Bee pollen
- Milk and cheese
- Bran flakes, rice bran

- Shellfish
- Brown rice
- Sardines
- Oatmeal, barley
- Sea vegetables
- Sprouts: lentils, mung beans, alfalfa, rye, wheat

BETA-CAROTENE, VITAMIN A AND D

Vitamin A, beta-carotene (the vitamin A found only in vegetables), and vitamin D go together for good health after 30. And there are more than 30 reasons why.

Beta Carotene Foods Reduce Cancer by 25% or More

One of the best cancer-fighters? All three, especially beta-carotene, help reduce your risk of cancer between 35 and 54, the high-risk years for cancer of the lungs, colon, rectum, pancreas, stomach, ovaries and breast, says the National Institute of Health. In one Harvard University study of 1,200 middle-aged Bostonites, those reporting the highest consumption of beta-carotene-rich vegetables[4] and fruits showed the lowest incidence of tumors. Even ex-smokers who added green-yellow vegetables reduced their risk of lung cancer by more than 25%.

The best sources of carotene (from excellent to good), says the National Cancer Institute, are carrots, squash, tomatoes, salads or leafy greens, dried fruits, fresh strawberries or melon, broccoli or Brussels sprouts.

What's the Difference Between Animal Vitamin A and Vegetable Vitamin A?

What's the difference between vitamin A and beta-carotene and how does vitamin D fit in? Vitamin A is the eyes, ears, nose and throat vitamin, and because of its role in blocking cancer, it also ranks as an antioxidant (so does beta-carotene). It builds post-30 resistance to infections, especially of the respiratory tract, keeps the outer layers of tissues and organs healthy, promotes general vitality, helps visual purple in the eye, counteracts night blindness and eyesight in general, and keeps your skin healthy and moist. Vitamin A is found in the same foods as carotene but in animal foods as well.

---

[4]If you're a gardener, look into the new USDA-developed super carrot called "A Plus" which provides 76% more caretene than the old-fashioned kind.

Improve Your Youthful Appearance in a Month or Less

Vitamin A even does you "youth-everlasting good turns" externally in the form of a prescription medication called Retinoic acid, researchers say at the Atlanta VA Medical Center. Vitamin A speeds up cell renewal and keeps skin fresher and younger-appearing and blocks wrinkling by tightening the skin. It also helps erase blemishes, liver spots and other age-related discolorations. A noticeable change usually occurs in three to four weeks.

Determine Your Vitamin A Needs and Don't Forget D

Vitamin A should be taken at meals with vitamin D. You can meet your daily needs with capsules of either vitamin A or beta-carotene (or both) supplying 5,000 (a base minimum) to 25,000 I.U. Or take 10,000 units of vitamin A and add a 5- to 10-mg. capsule of beta-carotene (the equivalent of 8,375 to 16,750 I.U. of A) for good anti-tumor insurance (smokers who are a higher risk should double this amount). Your state of health and your doctor can help you pinpoint your need. The more drugs you take or bad habits you have the more vitamin A and D you need. Careless cooking and food storage destroys the A and D, so do aspirin, alcohol and antacid, food additives and a wide range of prescription drugs, including those used for cholesterol-control foods.

How to Get Enough of "Both" A's from Meals and Snacks

Getting vitamin A at meals and between them is easy. Even a 1-ounce helping of sunflower seeds provides you 14 times the beta-carotene in a junkfood snack such as salted potato chips.

10 Ways Vitamin D Helps Slow Aging

Vitamin D occurs naturally with vitamin A in foods such as egg yolks and fish liver. It helps you assimilate vitamin A as well as calcium, phosphorus and magnesium to prevent bone softening, shrinkage, fracture and periodontal disease. A recent study of women over 50, for example, indicated that 40% had less than enough. Best and safest ways to get vitamin D is a daily dose of sunlight. Natural daylight increases the body's absorption of vitamin D. But vitamin D is developed and absorbed gradually (so don't shower too soon or remove the lipid layer on the skin that stores this vitamin D). Supplement to be on the safe side, too.

But enough of A and D is enough. More than 400 USP units of vitamin D by mouth daily increases susceptibility to arteriosclerosis, and sun-damaged older skin is more cancer-prone because skin's healing processes decline as you age. Best vitamin D foods are organ meats (liver, etc.), fatty fish, cod liver oil, milk, butter and egg yolks. Vitamin D deficiencies show up in muscular weakness and lack of vigor.

Top sources of vitamin A and beta-carotene

- Pumpkin
- Endive
- Olive oil (also supplies vitamin K and iron)
- Spaghetti squash
- Alfalfa
- Papaya
- Sweet potato
- Cantaloupe
- Butternut squash
- Apricots
- Zucchini squash
- Acorn squash
- Collard greens
- Carrots
- Chards
- Beet greens
- Spinach
- Broccoli
- Chayote squash
- Watermelon
- Hubbard squash
- Prunes
- Cherries
- Agar-agar (seaweed)
- Vitamin A and D supplements
- Beta-carotene supplements
- Green magma powder supplements (dried barley leaf)
- Wheat germ supplements

Top sources of vitamin D

- Egg yolks
- Meat
- Butter and margarine
- Fatty fish (sardines, tuna, salmon, mackerel)
- Dairy foods
- Nuts and seeds

Why You Need More Vitamin E After 40 to Fight These Four Age-Related Ills

"We're questioning the basic assumption that older people require smaller amounts of nutrients because their bodies are slowing down and because they're less active," says Dr. Jeffrey Blumberg, assistant director of government-funded Tufts University 1983 research project on aging. "While calorie requirements diminish, nutrient requirements are the same—even greater than they were. Getting more of certain nutrients may slow the aging process down," says Blumberg.

Why wait to be elderly to get those slowdown nutrients? At the top of the list you need more vitamin E. Why? Because it's your #1 nutritional defense against four if not more of the disorders that can get you after 40[5] if you don't watch out: heart disease, arthritis, stroke and cancer.

Six More Reasons You May Need More Vitamin E After 30

Where you find a sick heart, a stiff elbow, stroke or cancer, you're likely to find vitamin E deficiency. In one study by gerontologist Denham Harmon, M.D., Ph.D., of the University of Nebraska College of Medicine, cancer was noted after nine months in animals on a vitamin E-free, high-fat diet similar to that of the average affluent middle-aged American. Animals in a second group on the same diet but with a vitamin E supplement added did *not* show evidence of tumors until after 25 months—and the incidence was lower.

Vitamin E deficiency is often a cause of varicose veins, a circulatory condition that's likely to cramp your style if you're over 30 and eating from the wrong side of the menu. When unsightly cords pop out of your calves and ankles—that's a tipoff there's a weakness in the veins deep inside the leg muscles which carry up to 90% of the blood. It is the veins deep inside leg muscles which are first affected by pressure from your heart against the large pelvic veins. "What you are seeing in visible varicosities are nature's way of easing the burden of invisible varicosities deep within the leg . . . But superficial veins are too often disabled themselves in trying to carry this extra burden," says Philip H. Rakov, M.D., of the Department of Surgery at the State University of New York at Syracuse.

Even worse, the walls of veins may become inflamed in the condition known as phlebitis or a dark red solid mass of fibrin and blood cells may plug veins up in a more serious condition called thrombophlebitis, where

---

[5]Cancer and stroke were killers #9 and #5 respectively less than a century ago, now they,re #2 and 3. Heart disease, responsible for only 8% of all deaths in 1900, now account for 50% of all U.S. deaths. Other ills that make the list for you if you're over 40 include arthritis, plus a range of auto-immune maladies and diseases which may include scleroderma, lupus erythematosis, Parkinson's Disease and Alzheimer's Disease.

clots may break loose from the walls of the vein, be carried to the lungs or heart, where it may obstruct a crucial blood vessel and precipitate a heart attack.

Four Ways to Reverse Varicose Veins Without Drugs

Besides increased exercise, a minimum of sitting and a bulkier diet to prevent constipation, increased vitamin E can help. Vitamin E strengthens both the minor-league capillaries and the major-league deep veins, which in turn, tune up whole-body circulation, according to the Shute Foundation in London, Ontario, Canada, pioneers in vitamin E therapy.

Vitamin E and Fibrocystic Breast Disease

A second older-woman's disorder prevented and controlled by vitamin E is fibrocystis, the breast disease that isn't cancer. In one typical study, 600 mg. of vitamin E a day normalized disturbed hormone levels in the body that doctors believe lead to breast cyst formation in 80% of the victims. (Results are even better when sufferers abstain from caffeine, another contributing cause.)

Diabetes—which you are twice as likely to develop after 40 as you are after 20, says the Gerontology Research Center in Maryland, also responds to larger-than-drop-in-the-bucket amounts of vitamin E because it helps improve glycogen storage and normalizes insulin levels.

Vitamin E also keeps arteries clean, and clear of the fats and peroxides that promote clots and atherosclerosis. It lowers bad HDL cholesterol and raises LDL cholesterol by redistributing it, often in as little as two weeks. Doses of 600 I.U. or more a day often reduces the need for nitroglycerin where heart disorders have already existed.

The Magic Grain That Adds Vitamin E to All Your Meals

If you love wheat more than meat, getting E into your diet is easy. Wheat germ has 27 times more tocopherol (vitamin C) than steak. If you love salads, soybean oil has quadruple that amount. So won't any mixed well-balanced diet give you your minimum? Not unless you eat twice as well as the rest of us. The total daily average of vitamin E supplied by a typical American day at the table comes to only 7.4 mgs of vitamin E, which is about half the RDA, says the *American Journal of Clinical Nutrition*. Most nutritionists consider this amount extremely conservative. Don't skip supplements. But don't settle for ordinary supplements, either. Twelve to 15 mg.—the amount in most multivitamins—is the RDA, but 100 mg. is better.

Since vitamin E is, last but not least, an antioxidant, and a dose of at least 300 mg. a day is what it takes to block the formation of free radicals that induce age-related diseases, say researchers, taking vitamin E is a defensive step that may produce a marked decrease in cancer incidence as well as in that of other diseases.

Four Environmental Reasons to Boost Your Vitamin E Intake

There's another reason you need supplemental vitamin E—alcohol, chlorinated water, nitrates-containing foods such as processed lunch meats, bacon and a large variety of prescribed drugs, including hormone replacements, increase vitamin E needs. You also need more E if your polyunsaturated oil intake is up, says the American Medical Association. To benefit the most, take your E in the morning and your iron at night to prevent the neutralizing effect they may exert on each other. And take your E with vitamin C and selenium to extend vitamin E's antioxidant effect. Or, as an alternative, take it in a supplement formula that gives you at least one or more antioxidants such as SOD or selenium.

Top sources of vitamin E

- Olive oil
- Wheat germ, corn germ (liquids and flakes)
- Soybeans
- Vegetable and nut oils
- Nuts and seeds
- Broccoli
- Leafy salad greens
- Spinach, dandelion leaves
- Watercress
- Whole-grain cereals and breads
- Eggs
- Sea vegetables
- Sprouts: alfalfa, watercress, wheat
- Herb seasonings
- Vitamin E supplements
- Antioxidant formulas

CALCIUM

High-Calcium Foods Can Increase Your Life by 10 Years

Like to be a life-plusser and beat the national average of 73.8 years without taking youth serum? Do what the Tochipanese do. Residents of this tiny Japanese village live six to 10 years longer than the rest of us, says

Dr. Naga Ito, M.D., professor of nutrition at Japan's Sugiyama Women's College. This is becuase they consume twice as much vitamin C, vitamin A and vitamin B complex as we do, eat less and take more time doing it—but maybe, most important of all, they eat a lot more high-calcium foods, and get a lot more calcium-promoting exercise into their live-longer day. This may explain why so few of them are disabled by heart disease and bone disorders such as osteoporosis[6] that do us in.

What the National Institute on Aging Says About Calcium and Aging

"We used to think that all biological functions declined with age," says Dr. Edward L. Schneider, deputy director of the National Institute on Aging. "We now know that problems like osteoporosis are really diseases that we may be able to eliminate . . . This weakening of the bones with age that is a leading killer and crippler of older Americans is preventable by increasing calcium in the diet and encouraging lifelong physical activity." (Exercise promotes bone renewal. Studies indicate that older women getting the exercise equivalent of three sets of tennis can strengthen their skeletal bones to the equivalent of less active women ages 18–30.)

Why Women Need More Calcium than Men

According to 1984 studies by the National Institute on Aging, bone strength increases until the age of 30 to 35 in women. After that, it declines until menopause. Following menopause, female bone loss accelerates during the next three to seven years due to the decrease of estrogen levels and a tendency on the part of figure-conscious females to consume fewer calcium-rich foods. Calcium is one of the nutrients most frequently lacking in diets after 30. It is the most common mineral found in the body making up almost 2% of the weight of an adult. Ninety-nine percent of calcium is found in bones and teeth. Maintaining the remaining 1% in other compartments of your body is so important that if there is not enough calcium in the diet, it is removed from the bones. Osteoporosis is marked by a gradual loss of bone calcium and a weakening of skeletal strength. Increased ease of bone fracture, shrinking of body height and low backache may result from the loss of bone mass. Dowager's Hump and soft bones that fracture easily are common visible tipoffs. To make matters worse, women exercise less.

Older Men Benefit from Extra Calcium, Too

There are good reasons a 40-plus male should cut a rug and drink more milk, too. According to the *FDA Consumer*, increasing your calcium

---

[6]Are you an osteoporosis victim? Your doctor can administer a test to find out (see pages 9–10).

intake to a gram a day can reduce blood pressure by 6 to 10% in a matter of weeks. Calcium also lowers serum cholesterol by as much as 25%, speeds healing of broken bones, improves absorption of vitamin D and magnesium, makes the vitamin C you take go further, strengthens the heart muscle, prevents periodontal disease, rheumatoid arthritis and lowers stress. It even works better than aspirin and Midol to reduce pain, and even strengthens nails. (To tell at a glance if you need to bone up on calcium, check out your fingernails. Cracking or opaque white bands indicate calcium deficiency.)

Best Calcium Sources According to the American Heart Association

The American Heart Association recommends a daily intake of two or more cups of skim milk or skim-milk products. Although it has cholesterol—83 milligrams in an 8-ounce glass of whole milk—it has less than half the cholesterol of skinless chicken breast (79 mg.) or a 4-ounce piece of flounder (69 mg.). But milk's not the only source. Or the best.

Good Double-Value Calcium Foods

All-star calcium-rich common foods such as mackerel, flounder, salmon and sardines and uncommon ones such as sea vegetables and collards are double-value foods because they also provide life-extending nucleic acids (see Dr. Benjamin Frank's Longevity Diet, page 73). Exposing yourself to sunshine boosts your calcium retention, so does a dash of vinegar added to meat-bone soups. And there are two good roundabout ways to bone up—eat more greens. Scientists in Japan report that increased eating of greens with vitamin K reduces the loss of calcium from bones— often by 50%. Good sources of K include dark greens, broccoli and lettuce, and drink less coffee. Caffeine is linked to loss of calcium. In one recent study, 300 mg. of caffeine—the amount in two to three cups of brewed coffee—doubled the amount of calcium that was lost in the urine compared to drinking non-caffeined drinks.

Mineral-Taker's Tips

Calcium and magnesium should be taken together, two parts of calcium to one or two parts of magnesium. The RDA is 800 mg. but a good post-30 intake, especially for women who need it most, is 1,500 to 2,000 mg. a day.[7] (This is the amount now recommended by the National Institute of Health.) The best way to get both is probably calcium orotate taken at bedtime with 500 mg. of magnesium orotate. Calcium carbonate

---

[7]More than 2,000 mg. a day can be risky if you have a personal or family history of kidney stones. Ask your doctor about the simple lab test that detects this susceptibility and be sure to drink 4 to 8 glasses of liquid a day as stone-prevention strategy.

which provides more calcium per tablet than other forms is the best second choice. After that, the three best choices are calcium chloride, calcium lactate or calcium gluconate. Better yet, buy a calcium-plus supplement that provides calcium in more than one form.

Can you get the calcium you need from food? Life-plussers like the Tochipanese get theirs from unrefined, healthy food—maybe you can, too. But don't bet on it. The older you are the less calcium your body absorbs— and the more you cut calories, the more you reduce calcium. A deficiency of vitamin D, too much vitamin C or protein, alcohol, diuretics or a heavy antacid habit draw calcium from the bones, too, and keep levels low by blocking uptake. Still, food *is* the best place to start.

Along with cutting a rug or playing tennis to promote your post-30 calcium reserves, here's an easy way to get more calcium into your live-longer meals using everyday foods. One item on the excellent list is equal to three on the fair list.

Excellent sources

- 1 cup any flavor yogurt
- 1 cup milk (skim, lowfat or whole)
- 8 oz. milk shake
- ½ 10-inch pizza
- ½ cup mackerel or salmon
- 2¾ oz. tin herring

Good sources

- 1 bean-and-cheese burrito
- 3 pancakes made with milk
- 1 serving any frozen entree with cheese
- 1 cup ice milk or frozen yogurt
- 2 oz. (1½-inch cube) any hard cheese (except Swiss)
- 1 cup kale, chard, turnip, collard or mustard greens

Fair sources

- ⅓ cup almonds
- 1 cup baked beans
- 1 cup cocoa
- 1 fudgsicle
- ½ cup oysters
- 1 cup broccoli or okra

Top sources of calcium

- Sardines
- Lentils (red are richer than green)
- Wheat germ
- Pistachio nuts
- Brazil nuts
- Sunflower seeds
- Cottage cheese
- Watercress
- Whole-grain bread, whole-wheat cereal
- Chickpeas, dried
- Dandelion greens
- Kale
- Rutabaga
- Cabbage
- Soyflour
- Artichoke
- Sesame seeds
- Soybeans
- Blackstrap molasses
- Filberts
- Cashews
- Bean curd (tofu)
- Shrimp
- Lavender Gem and Blood oranges
- All tropical fruits
- Bentonite (edible clay), a nutritional supplement
- Mugwort, an herbal supplement and tea
- Unrefined 100% cane sugar (see *Mail Sources*)
- Calcium supplements including bonemeal, oystershell, eggshell and dolomite

MAGNESIUM

Running low on magnesium in midlife can be risky business.[8] And if your diet's just average, research indicates, you're probably averaging 236 mg. to 270 mg. a day—100% short of your normal needs. Even shorter if your needs *aren't* normal.

Why Low Magnesium Levels Increase the Risk of Heart Disease

According to the American Medical Association, 40% of all fatal heart attacks may be caused by coronary spasms caused in turn by magnesium deficiency. The hearts of attack victims often contain 10 to 35% less magnesium than the hearts of those who die from other causes, says the American Society for Magnesium Research. "Animal studies show a low magnesium-high blood pressure link, and magnesium may regulate the flow of calcium to the muscle cells lining arteries. If magnesium is depleted by stress, cells overload with calcium and blood vessels contract, producing hypertension," they report.

The Canadian National Research Council Advises More Magnesium for the Active

Magnesium is central to energy metabolism after 30. It's one of the body's most important nutrients because of adenosine triphosphate (ATP). Energy is produced in the body when ATP releases phosphorus. Without magnesium, the chemical reaction just doesn't come off. An intense physical activity like long-distance swimming can reduce magnesium levels sharply in just 60 minutes and keep them low for as long as three months, says the Canadian National Research Council. Magnesium also helps prevent kidney stones, gallstones and calcium deposits, says Dr. Hans Selye of McGill University in Toronto.

Six Benefits of More Magnesium

Magnesium is also an anti-stress nutrient, an essential for carbohydrate metabolism, muscle function and metabolism of other live-longer minerals such as calcium. It contributes to bone growth, acid/alkaline

---

[8]University of California at Davis studies show that a mild magnesium depletion can reduce birthweight of newborns by 30%.

balance and the normal blood sugar levels. More important, it prevents mental confusion and disorientation, according to the National Research Council. Getting your adult daily dose of calcium (the amount in a bowl of shredded wheat with skim milk and wheat germ on top) may be a hedge against such brain-fade disorders as Alzheimer's disease which afflicts 3 million Americans. According to new research at the University of Mexico, a shortage of magnesium along with folic acid and B-complex can lead to early senility.

Seven Magnesium Snacks That Boost Youthful Vigor

Magnesium occurs in most plant foods with the richest common sources being—nuts; beans; legumes; whole grains; greeny, leafy vegetables like spinach, kale and beet greens. (It's also found in chocolate.) Cooking can deplete the amount you get and raw foods are richer than processed ones. One example? Magnesium levels in refined sugar are only 2 ppm. In unsulphured molasses they are 5,206 ppm.

Take the Amount That's Healthiest for You

Magnesium should be taken in the right ratio with other minerals. A supplement providing 800 mg. of calcium and 400 mg. magnesium is a good bet. And if you need anti-stress help, you might heed the advice of Dr. Carl Pfeiffer of Princeton, New Jersey's Brain-Bio Center and take a supplement that provides 500 mg. of magnesium oxide and 1,000 mg. of calcium orotate at bedtime. Magnesium is depleted by antibiotics, antacids, diuretics, alcohol, too much protein or calcium, menstruation and stress, including pregnancy and intense exercise.

Best sources of magnesium

- Almonds and almond butter
- Brazil nuts
- Wheat bran and wheat germ
- Dried fruits
- Filberts
- Brown rice
- Millet
- Oatmeal
- Sesame seeds
- Cashew nuts
- Corn, fresh
- Walnuts

- Pecans
- Sunflower seeds
- Nut butters
- Sea vegetables
- Seafood
- Soyfoods (tofu, tempeh, miso, etc.)
- Chocolate and cocoa
- Sprouts: alfalfa, watercress, soybeans
- Brewer's yeast
- Soy sauce
- Magnesium supplements
- Calcium-magnesium mineral supplements
- Dolomite supplements

SELENIUM, ZINC, BHT, SOD, B-15 (ANTIOXIDANTS)

Trace Minerals Help You Win the Bad Habit Battle

If you're 40 or more and you haven't gotten a perfect score on your youth potential (page 8), now's the time you begin to feel the effects of how you've treated your body, says Dr. John Rowe of Harvard University Medical School. "Keep physically active, stop smoking and switch to a low-fat diet."

If you're having trouble doing all three of those things, a few antioxidants can protect you from yourself and help you in your time-clock battle. They can even help if you've covered all those bases[9] because antioxidants are anti-cancer, anti-autoimmune system nutrients.

According to National Academy of Sciences funded studies, the mortality rate of 35- to 74-year-old white males is twice as high in the southeast United States as it is the upper middle-west, because the soil and water there has smaller amounts of the life-lengthening antioxidant trace minerals chromium, selenium and zinc as well as major minerals such as magnesium.

---

[9]Even is you have *no* bad habits, antioxidants protect you from people who do. According to a survey by the Naitonal Institute of Environmental and Health Sciences, people who live with one smoker face a cancer risk 1.4 times higher than those who don't. The risk is 2.3 times higher for those who live with two smokers and 2.6 times greater for those who live with three or more smokers. The risk includes leukemia and breast, cervix as well as lung cancer.

Antioxidants Prevent Post-30 Body Rust

Antioxidants, says Dr. C. Wayne Callaway of the Mayo Clinic are substances that protect other substances from being burned up by oxygen, preventing a sort of internal "body rust" which leads to disease. In the body, antioxidants protect your reserves of vitamin A (itself an antioxidant) and polyunsaturated fatty acids and prevent premature aging of cells.

There are lots of body rust-busters—vitamin A and C qualify. So does beta-carotene along with B-15 (also known as pangamic acid or "DMG," or N-Dimethylglycine), and the bioflavonoids—vitamin E and zinc. Amino acids and niacin and niacinamide even make rejuvenation lists such as the American Geriatric Society's, and newcomers such as SOD and BHT are essentials in the view of UCLA gerontologist Roy Walford.

Which to take and which to forget? That depends on how much you need and how much you get already from your daily diet. It also depends on your health. If it's not so good, take more. The list of life-shortening conditions improved by antioxidants include cancer (new evidence from the University of Knopio, Finland, indicates low blood levels of selenium, vitamin E and vitamin A increase your risk of developing that cancer), arthritis, diabetes, hypertension and reduced immune response.

Big Magic Comes in Minimum Doses

Small as it sounds, just 50 to 100 micrograms of selenium[10] could be a time-clock stopper. Gerontologists such as Dr. Richard Passwater recommends 50 to 200 mcg. a day to keep the immune system healthy enough to resist the disease of aging. That amount added to the diets of laboratory rats increased their life span 14%. In man, that corresponds to a life extension of 15 years.

The Miracle of Selenium

Similarly, a selenium-rich diet (more whole grains, brewer's yeast, fermented foods and sea vegetables) is the reason breast cancer in Japan is just half of what it is in the United States, according to the Third International Symposium on Selenium in Biology and Medicine. Selenium also helps prevent diabetes retinopathy plus senile and muscular degeneration (two major causes of blindness). It slows the development of high blood pressure and rheumatoid arthritis, improves energy and alertness and blocks stress.

Selenium helps protect your post-40's health from toxic chemicals in drinking water such as asbestos, chlorine, fluoride, nickel and mercury

---

[10]Selenium levels in water, soil and plants vary as much as 200%. They are lower on both coasts and highest in the interior states.

which increase the risk of cancer and heart disease, as well as cadmium found in coffee and tea and in grains, rice and sugar when they are refined, says the Foundation for Alternative Cancer Therapies. Selenium also helps prevent chromosome damage in tissues that cause birth defects, and a 100 mcg. tablet of selenium a day is often all that's needed to eliminate the low-back pain blues. There is no RDA for selenium, but a 50 to 100 mcg. tablet a day is a good intake—more can be toxic.

Too Little Zinc Leads to Rapid Aging

After selenium, zinc is number two on your life-extending antioxidant shopping list. Zinc is a constituent of nearly 100 human enzymes involved in all the body's major metabolic processes. It's a must in activating antioxidant amounts of vitamin A and transporting them from your liver to your bloodstream. With a zinc deficiency goes a vitamin A deficiency and with that double-trouble debt—goes premature aging. Zinc is a must for decay-free teeth and resistance to bacteria and viral infections, especially when coupled with anti-viral vitamin C. Take zinc-C lozenges when you feel your next cold coming on.

Zinc can save your skin in the second half of life. According to the Proceedings of the National Academy of Sciences, "Experiments in which mice were given diets with different levels of zinc demonstrated that those on very low levels gradually lost weight and many of them died. Half of the animals on zinc-deficient diets showed skin changes, especially on tail and paws. They also had diarrhea and acrodermatitis, an inflammatory condition of the skin. None of these symptoms appeared in the animals given plenty of zinc."

Tipoffs That You're Suffering Zinc Deficiency

Zinc deficiency can produce anything from canker sores to B.O. to halitosis, from a pain in the knee or hip to a poor immune response and diminished taste perception. The RDA for zinc is 15 mg., too low to protect yourself from any age-related disease you've already got or don't want. Thirty milligrams is a better bet, especially taken in a supplement formation that includes a few other antioxidants such as selenium and A. (Chelated forms are better absorbed. Doses up to 150 mg. daily are considered safe.)

After zinc, think SOD. Superoxide dismutase (SOD) is a water-soluble protein found throughout your body, especially in the liver, red blood cells and bony tissues. Studies at the Gerontology Research Center in Baltimore showed that animals with the longest life spans had the highest nutritional levels of SOD in their bodies. Those with the shortest life spans had the least amount present.

What the Metabolic Research Foundation Says About SOD

Dr. Harold Manner of the Metabolic Research Foundation who uses drug-free therapy to treat cancer, arthritis and rheumatism, says, "SOD should be a definite part of the supplement program for anyone fearful of cancer."[11] And according to gerontologists Dr. Hans Kugler and Richard Passwater, SOD should occur normally in the body in amounts 100,000 times greater than the free radicals it fights—but when aging sets in it doesn't. To compensate for dipping reserves of SOD, take tablets of SOD (250 mg. daily) or freeze-dried liver tablets.

A Good Food Additive That Fights Aging

As for BHT (Butylated Hyphoxyltolulene) this new-to-the-health-fight-after-30 antioxidant does what the other anti-body-rust nutrients do and then some, says Dr. Walford, if you want to feel safe. Among other findings—new research indicates 2 grams a day of BHT helps deactivate the two major forms of herpes virus which afflict 5 to 20 million adults. Herpes occurs when the immune response is poor and BHT improves your immune response. BHT is sold in supplements (250 mg. a day is a protective dose). It's also used as a food preservative in a wide variety of processed foods.

Scientific Studies Say B-15 Improves Your Immunity

Another immune booster antioxidant not to be missed is B-15, better known as DMG (dimethylglycine)—the vitamin that's really an adaptogen (like ginseng), a substance contained in calcium pangamate which scientific studies at the University of South Carolina conclude helps strengthen immunity. When researchers gave 20 healthy patients DMG tablets, the results were a fourfold jump in production of protective antibodies. And when taken by patients with immune systems affected by diabetes and sickle cell anemia, B-15 doubled the immune responses.

Russian research indicates that taking B-15 increases the supply of oxygen in your bloodstream and improves the uptake of oxygen into all the body tissues. Also, it helps detoxify oxygen-consuming pollutants from the blood, relieves the symptoms of cardiovascular conditions and the discomfort of angina and normalizes cholesterol levels in the blood. According to the world-renowned B-15 researcher Yakov Shpirt, "Calcium pangamate (B-15) is a potent stimulant in the control of aging." It even fights cancer. At least one Russian experiment on record credits B-15 significantly reduced both incidence and onset of induced mammary tumors in young rats.

U.S. doctors on DMG's side include gerontologist Dr. Richard Passwa-

---

[11]The drug derived from superoxide dismutase, orgotein, is currently used in Europe for relief of arthritis and other joint diseases.

ter who prescribes B-15 as a "second wind" power supplement for the Washington Redskins, and super-energy diet doctor Robert Atkins, who prescribes B-15 as a pick-me-up: "When none of the other vitamins work, B-15 can turn a patient's energy picture around." Fifty to 100 mg. is a good daily dose.

Why You Need Supplements to Get Antioxidants into Your Diet

Antioxidant trace minerals, unlike essential vitamins and minerals, are not easy to get from diet alone. The best sources are the least accessible. (If you ate beets grown on Soviet Georgian soil, or peaches grown in Georgia, USA, or had access to Hunza's glacial waters, you'd never have to give antioxidants a second thought.)

Even if you don't have any serious health problems now—supplementing with E and C or adding two out of five antioxidants discussed once a week is not a bad plan, along with a varied diet that concentrates on the best of the most age-related foods.

Top sources of antioxidants

- Selenium—fish and shellfish, fruits and vegetables (especially onions), beef liver, beef kidney, lamb or pork kidney, organ meats, muscle meats, dairy products, grains and cereals, selenium-fortified brewer's yeast. Selenium tablets and capsules.
- Zinc—oysters, herring, clams, liver, wheat germ or bran, brewer's yeast, pumpkin seeds, eggs, powdered milk, whole milk, yogurt, all whole grains. Zinc tablets and lozenges.
- SOD—fresh or freeze-dried beef and calves liver, sea vegetables, yeast, pollen and propolis. SOD is the prime ingredient in the arthritis prescription drug orgotein. SOD/liver supplements.
- BHT—a preservative in processed foods, sold in tablets/capsules and some antioxidant formulas.
- B-15—brewer's and nutritional yeast, whole grains, pollen, alfalfa seeds. B-15 supplements.

HERBS

The Secret of the World's Oldest Young People

What's the USSR's Georgian region got—besides cleaner air and better borsht—that makes it a longevity hot spot? Soil and water that's richer in life-extending ingredients, especially selenium and zinc, according to the International Selenium Symposium—and that means healthier herbs to eat, drink and season food with.

When it comes to a something-for-nothing-fountain-of-youth food, nothing compares to herbs, even if yours aren't Soviet-grown. They are nature's only next-to-no-calories, low-in-sodium, no-fat, fiber-rich, sugar-free foods. Maybe parsley and rosehips don't top anybody's list of longevity essentials, but if you've taken care of foods and supplements, then beat-the-clock workouts come next.

A Good No-Calorie Source of Staying Young Minerals

Herbs[12] provide both major and the minor minerals—especially the trace elements such as copper, zinc and selenium that program your system to prevent disease. A typical mid-lifer's supermarket-dependent diet is likely to be low in these elements because they are lost when food is refined for extended shelf life.

When it comes to trace minerals, there is magic in a minimum dose. (A Hostess Twinkie contains no selenium, but one hefty parsley and endive salad gives you all the selenium (50 mcg.) you need to provide selenium's time-fighting effect.) And a little goes a long way and can be optimally beneficial in affecting your body's slowly slowing-down process. An herb weed such as Nettle contains iron, copper and manganese in proportions that are needed to build blood, which is why it is still considered a reliable RX for anemia. As a bonus, it's rich in blood-enriching chlorophyll.

Fight Bad Breath, Arthritis and Osteoporosis with Parsley Tea

Plain, everyday parsley, for example—a member of the carrot-par-snip-celery family—has been used for centuries in treating such ills of aging as arthritis, cancer and hair loss. Parsley seeds can be chewed to better an on-the-fritz digestive tract or sweeten up pizza-eater's breath, and parsley provides more calcium and osteoporosis-preventative vitamin K and more vitamin A than any other leafy green.

10 Benefits of Ginseng

Or consider ginseng, the most famous rejuvenator of them all. It detoxifies the blood; feeds and stimulates the brain, the endocrine glands and the nervous system; aids digestion and assimilation of vitamins and minerals, prolongs strength and stamina, sharpens reflexes and improves mental concentration and balance, says the Cancer Research Institute. And Japanese researchers have recently reported that the saponius in Asian ginseng protects liver cells from damage when exposed to toxic chemicals.

---

[12]What qualifies as an herb besides the teas you know and sip? Botanically speaking, spices and seasoning such as cinnamon qualify, so do potatoes, tomatoes and cabbage. And if you have an occasional nip, have one that contains 130 different herbs—chartreuse liqueur.

Rejuvenate Your Senses with Herbs

They won't work miracles and they don't produce overnight reults, but along with alfalfa, parsley, dandelion, licorice and gotu kola, they have their own roll-back-the-years, get-your-ball-rolling-again effect. Depression, for example, may be better treated with herbs in tea or tincture (oil) form. Peppermint soaked in mint oil is a safe brain perk, too, according to the International Flavors and Fragrances Institute. And French psychoanalyist Andre Virel recommends pure vanilla extract, a well-known stimulant of the limbic system: "Cells that do our smelling are linked up to the limbic system," says Virel, "and that's the part of the 'old brain' that controls feelings, moods and memory."

Herb Tea, the Antacid Alternative

And if the problem is post-40's flatulence, the answer—besides eliminating sugar, increasing exercise and skipping over-the-counter antacids (they worsen hyperacidity and deplete your calcium reserves),—suggests herbal expert Jeanne Rose, is chamomile, comfrey leaf, fennel seed, peppermint and thyme. Grind them small, mix them up and drink a cup or two from the tea you make after each meal. Sage and rosemary, Rose says, stimulate the secretion of bile which is essential in the digestion of fats, another gas-making situation if the bile is not provided in large enough quantity, and the herbs contain essential oils that promote digestion.

Or try Brazilian Herb Tea, for example. Maybe it isn't the "treasure of the Incas," that the Indians have claimed for thousands of years, says Utal herbalist Dr. John Heinerman, but if it improves any one of the five age-related conditions it's said to, such as arthritis, asthma, diabetes, cancer and herpes, it's worth a sip. Even if it doesn't, it's rich in antioxidant trace minerals—and, unlike coffee and tea, it's free of gastric irritants such as caffeine, and carcinogens such as tannin, both of which reduce your intake of iron and vitamin C.

Eat the Flowers to Reverse PMS, Poor Sight, Vitamin Deficiencies

And don't forget flowers are healthy herbs, too. Dried, you can turn them into a cup of rejuvenation tea or use them fresh as edible garnishes for soups and stews. Mums, violets, rosebuds, unscented geraniums and dandelion buds provide longevity vitamins A, C, D, iron and calcium—and some are Mother Nature's sources of female hormones that are helpful in treating PMS, vision problems and discouraging superficial facial hair.

What belongs in your arsenal for herbal renewal? Take a look at the list that follows and take your pick—but choose at least six to use regularly as teas, seasonings or ingredients. Herbs can be taken in tablets, capsules and liquid supplement form—singly or in combination. A good forget-menot way to use more herbs? Always add one to the pot or plate whenever you cook a meal.

Top sources of herbs

- Vitamin A: Alfalfa, Dandelion, Okra, Violets
- Vitamin C: Burdock seed, Calendula, Capsicum, Coltsfoot, Elderberries, Oregano, Paprika, Parsley, Rosehips, Watercress
- Vitamin D: Watercress, Dandelion buds
- Calcium: Arrowroot, Irish moss, Dulse, Camomile, Chives, Coltsfoot, Comfrey, Dandelion root, Alfalfa, Parsley, Nettle, Borage, Sorrel, Okra, Boneset, Silica
- Iron &   Burdock root, Meadowsweet, Mullein, Nettle,
  Vitamin K: Parsley, Alfalfa, Strawberry and Raspberry Leaves, Watercress, Dandelion
- Magnesium: Bladderwrack, Carrot tops, Dandelion, Kale, Meadowsweet, Mullein, Okra, Parsley, Peppermint, Walnut Leaves, Watercress, Wintergreen
- Potassium: Birch bark, Carrot tops, Camomile, Comfrey, Dandelion, Fennel, Mullein, Nettle, Parsley, Peppermint, Primrose Flowers, Savory, Watercress, Yarrow
- Antioxidants, Ginseng, Alfalfa, Bladderwrack, Dandelion
  Including   leaves, Sesame seed, Watercress, Broccoli, Celery
  Vitamin E: leaves

Sources: American Herb Trade Association
                 Herb Research Foundation
                 American Herb Foundation
                 Herbal Gram Newsletter

ACTION PLAN FOR STAYING YOUNG: NUTRIENTS GUIDE

Here are the nutrients you need and the amounts you need them in, according to the Food and Nutrition Board of the National Academy of Sciences:

Calories	2050-2400	1600-1800
Nutrients	*Men*	*Women*
Protein (g.)	56	44

Nutrients	Men	Women
Vitamin A (I.U.)	5,000	4,000
Vitamin E (I.U.)	15	12
Vitamin D (I.U.)	400	400
Vitamin C (mg.)	60	60
Folic Acid (mcg.)	400	400
Niacin (mg.)	16	13
Riboflavin (mg.)	1.4	1.2
Thiamine (mg.)	1.2	1
Vitamin B-6 (mg.)	2.2	2
Vitamin B-12 (mcg.)	3	3
Calcium (mg.)	800	800
Magnesium (mg.)	350	300
Zinc (mg.)	15	15

In the opinion of the best alternative medical experts and nutritionists, this doesn't begin to provide any life-extending benefits. And it's doubtful whether it's enough to meet ordinary needs.[13] That means it's up to you and your doctor to decide what a better intake might be.

If you'd like a second opinion after that or if you'd like to be referred to a nutritionist in your area, write American Association of Nutritional Consultants, 1641 E. Sunset Road, B-117, Las Vegas, Nevada 89119, or a member of the American Dietician's Association (members are listed with an R.D. after their names under "dieticians" in your yellow pages).

TIPS FOR VITAMIN-TAKERS

1. You can be a better consumer, spend your supplement money more wisely and be more aware of what you are putting into your body by learning how to read a label.

• The first thing to look for is how many tablets contain what potency. (Does the label say: "One tablet will supply the following amounts," or does it say "Three tablets daily will supply the following amounts"?). If the nutrient name is followed by a statement in parentheses, it indicates the source of the nutrient, and the actual amount is the full amount as stated on the label. No parentheses? The potency in the compound will be much less.

• Most nutrient contents appear as milligrams or micrograms. They are measurements of weight, and you cannot compare weights

---

[13]The RDA is based on the needs of a healthy population and does not take physical or emotional stress or unusual lifestyle circumstances or the aging process into consideration. In addition, the RDA is directed at population groups in America, minimizing the effects that local environments have on nutrient needs.

of different nutrients. You can compare the amount of vitamin C in one preparation with the C in another, but not vitamin C with vitamin B-1. Weights are in metric form and the three most common are: 1 grain (gr.) equal to 64.8 milligrams (mg.); 1 milligram equal to 1,000 micrograms (mcg.); 1 gram (g.) is equal to 15.43 grains, or 1,000 milligrams equal 1 million micrograms.

• Oil-soluble vitamins (A, F, D) are measured in International Units (I. U.). The I.U. is a measurement of effect, meaning that a certain amount of the nutrient causes a reaction in the body. I.U. of one vitamin cannot be compared to the I.U. of any other vitamin.

2. What's best—tablets, capsules, powders, liquid or time-released? Experiment. If oil-based A, E and D upset your stomach, try dry or buffered forms. If you hate to take big pills, take powder or small spoonfuls of vitamins in higher potency forms. Time-released is good if you empty your bowels in 18 to 24 hours. If it's 6 hours or less, you'll lose a lot.

3. Water-soluble vitamins remain in the body about six hours, so take them three times a day. (And wash them down with water, not coffee or tea. Caffeine drinks reduce the absorption of nutrients by 45%.)

4. Supplements are organic substances which should be taken with foods for best absorption—especially the water-soluble B complex and C, which are excreted rapidly in the urine. If this is not convenient, take half with breakfast, half with dinner. If you must take all your vitamins at once, do it with your largest meal of the day. If you're a forgetter, use your fridge. Keeping vitamins and fruit juices side by side as an instant sip-and-supplement reinforcer.

5. Adjust your dosage to your weight. The smaller and lighter you are the less your need and vice versa.

6. Change your timetable if you have to take medications,[14] too. Drugs should be taken two hours before or after meals to minimize the loss of nutrients. Even so you stand to lose a few. Here are some of the commonest prescription drugs, what they deplete from the body and which foods help you compensate for the loss.

---

[14]Take them safely. Write for a free pamphlet with up-to-date facts on over-the-counter and prescription drugs from Schering-Plough Corp. Information Services, 2000 Galloping Hill Road, Kenilworth, New Jersey 07033.

THE AGING EFFECT OF COMMON MEDICATIONS

Drug	Aging Effect . . .	To Prevent Increase. . .
Oral contraceptive pills (birth control)	Deficiency of folic acid, vitamins B6, B12 and C; iron, copper and zinc	Leafy green vegetables, sea vegetables such as dulse, whole grains and organ meats (kidney, liver)
Antibiotics (Bacterial infections)	Vitamin B complex deficiency	Yogurt, sprouts, nutritional yeast
Aspirin (Arthritis and long term use)	Deficiency of vitamin C and calcium; skin inflammation[15]	Citrus fruits, milk products, salads
Antihistamines (Allergies and colds)	Vitamin B complex deficiency	Whole grains, green vegetables, eggs, liver
Water pills (High blood pressure control and dieting)	Potassium deficiency	Bananas, parsley, lean meat
Cortisone (Arthritis)	Vitamin C deficiency	Citrus and tropical fruits, greens
Cholesterol control drugs	Vitamin K deficiency	Cabbage, tomatoes, leafy greens, liver
Antacids (Upset stomach)	Magnesium deficiency	Whole grains, nuts, dark leafy greens
Hormone drugs (Menopause)	Deficiency of folic acid and vitamin E	Leafy green vegetables, liver and whole grains
Blood sugar reducing drugs (Diabetes)	Vitamin B12 deficiency	Meats, brewer's yeast, eggs, sea vegetables such as kelp

---

[15]New research at Harvard Medical School indicated that 5 to 10% of all cases of chronic and acute hives are caused by aspirin.

Drug	Aging Effect...	To Prevent Increase...
Drugs for treating peptic ulcers	Vitamin K deficiency, B12 deficiency	Egg yolks, leafy greens, cauliflower
Gout-treating drugs	Deficiency of vitamin C and thiamine	Citrus fruits, whole grains
Alcohol	B12, folic acid, iron, zinc, magnesium, calcium deficiency	Nutritional yeast, liver, brown rice, whole-grain cereal, pumpkin and sesame seeds, wheat germ
Anti-inflammatory and other non-narcotic analgesics	Folic acid, vitamin C, iron deficiency	Citrus fruits, root vegetables, salad greens
Anticoagulants	Deficiency of folic acid	Leafy greens, sea vegetables, liver powder
Gastrointestinal drugs	Vitamin A, D and folic acid deficiency	Fish liver, oils, sea vegetables, eggs
Tranquilizers	Deficiency of riboflavin (B2)	Yogurt, yeast, sprouts
Air pollutants	All vitamins	Fish liver, oil, dairy products, leafy green vegetables, wheat germ oil, nuts and seeds
Arsenic and Arsenicals	Deficiency of vitamin A, PABA	PABA, liver, wheat germ, fatty fish, nutritional yeast, molasses
Carbon monoxide	Vitamin C deficiency	Fresh fruits and vegetables
Fluoride	Vitamin C deficiency	Fresh fruits and vegetables
Chlorine (In tap water and swimming pools)	Vitamin E deficiency	Wheat germ, corn oil, whole wheat
Coffee, soft drinks (Containing caffeine)	Deficiency of B1, inositol, biotin, potassium, zinc; reduces calcium and iron assimilation	Wheat germ and bran, brown rice, nutritional yeast, beets, blackstrap molasses

Drug	Aging Effect...	To Prevent Increase...
Tobacco	Vitamin C, B1, calcium, phosphorus, B complex, folic acid	Fresh fruits, vegetables, dairy products, leafy greens

Sources

- American Dietetic Association.
- American Psychiatric Association (7 to 10% of outpatient and 20 to 40% of inpatient psychiatric cases are caused by medical conditions or drugs, says the APA).
- Daphne A. Roe, M.D. *Handbook of Interactions of Selected Drugs and Nutrients Among Patients.*

4

Exercises for
Prolonging Your Life

THE LIFE-EXTENDING BENEFITS OF EXERCISING

1. High-calorie burn-off
2. Cardiovascular conditioner
3. Muscular endurance
4. Muscular strength
5. Flexibility/figure shaping
6. Balance/Posture
7. Weight loss/Weight control
8. Sociability
9. Stress reduction

- Approximate. This varies depending on intensity and body weight. Based on criteria by President's Council on Physical Fitness, American Health Association and Aerobics Institute in Dallas.

- Every fitness routine outlined in this book provides Live-Longer benefits. To determine which exercise is best for what—match the numbers which follow it with the numbers in the key above.

STAY YOUNG EXERCISES

Age cannot "wither" nor custom "stale," as the saying goes. At least it gets less of a foot in the door if you exercise. All it takes is 30 minutes three times a week.

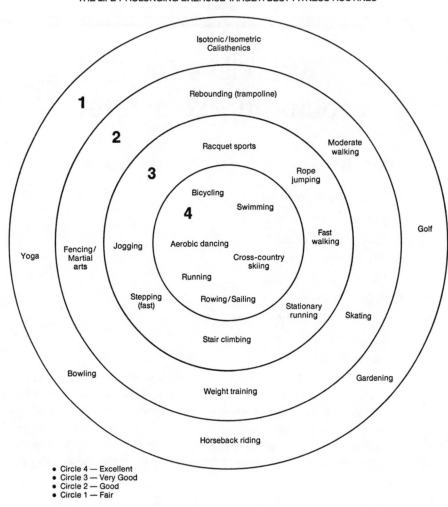

THE LIFE-PROLONGING EXERCISE TARGET: BEST FITNESS ROUTINES

- Circle 4 — Excellent
- Circle 3 — Very Good
- Circle 2 — Good
- Circle 1 — Fair

Figure 4-1

And don't sit it out to be on the safe side if you're on the wrong side of 30 or 40. According to Dr. Raymond Harris, founder of the Albany Center for the Study of Aging, "the risks of *not* exercising are a greater hazard to an older person's health than exercising."[1]

Some of exercise's goods and services you already know about are— its ability to improve the efficiency of your heart (exercisers have one-third fewer heart attacks than non-exercisers), lower cholesterol, increase muscular strength and energy and improve the uptake of calcium by the bones, not to mention what working out does for weight, skin tone, sleepless nights and post-40's stress. "Excessive reactions to stress have been shown, among other effects, to depress the actions of the immune system, setting the stage for a variety of ills," says Dr. Kenneth R. Pelletier of the department of psychiatry at the University of California at San Francisco.

But here are a few of the goods you may *not* know about that you get when you go for that spin or swim—

• Exercising aids arthritis sufferers by preventing muscles from becoming weak and joints stiff. (*Note*: When there is active inflammation from rheumatoid arthritis, exercise should be curtailed.)

• Improves diabetic recovery by promoting insulin production and better use of glucose by the body.

• Reduces depression and anxiety better than drugs.

• Exercise reduces the risk of auto-immune diseases such as cancer, which peak between 45 and 65. Scientists at Japan's Labor Science Research Institute discovered when they divided cancer-susceptible mice into two groups, the first got plenty of exercise running on special wheels inside their cages; the rest were confined to cages without a "gym." Results? Sixty percent of the sedentary mice developed liver tumors, compared to less than 24% of the active mice.

• Being a busy body slows down middle-age spread by keeping pounds in the right place. Without exercise, even the fit turn to fat with age. Changes in metabolism and hormones lead to changes in muscle tone, says Dr. Kenneth Minaker, assistant professor at Harvard Medical School. The result: muscle turns to fat and deposits increase in the stomach area and decrease in arms, legs and chest. "A 140-pound sergeant in the army might still weigh 140 pounds 20 years later, but he probably won't be able to buckle his belt." Daily exercise prevents degeneration of muscle tissue.

• If you're already thin with only one chin, gravity-reversing exercise helps you reap one more reward—according to Dr. Hamilton Hall, assistant professor of surgery at the University of Toronto, gravity can squeeze the fluids in the discs of the spine (discs return to normal while you sleep).

---

[1]Women take this to heart more than men. Women are 18% more active than men, says the National Family Opinion Survey. For every 22.4 million American males who are fresh-water fishing, there are 22.4 million women who are swimming.

The disc fluid gradually dries out with age which is why older people appear to shrink as they age. Anti-gravity workouts such as gymnastics, yoga and calisthenics prevent this teeny-weeny effect.

• Exercise keeps you in "nitrogen balance" as you age. Losing more nitrogen than you are taking in puts you in negative nitrogen balance. (Nitrogen comes from the amino acids that make up body protein.) Negative balance means your body is using more protein to maintain and repair cells than your diet is providing. That protein eventually will be drawn from body protein reserves including your spine and jaw bone. Exercise helps the body retain its protein reserves.

• Your older but better brain benefits when you keep your body moving, says Dr. Richard E. Dustman, a research psychologist at the VA Hospital in Salt Lake City, Utah. In his study of post-50 sedentary males put on exercise regimes, out of eight mental tests, including reaction time and short-term memory, only the group that did the most aerobic exercise (brisk walking) improved significantly in six of them. Their brain gains matched their improved oxygen intake. No-memory-loss exercisers also had more intact cardiovascular systems. The brain, like the heart, works best with plenty of oxygen.

• "Regular exercise produces very small charges of electricity which help remineralize bones, making them hard, dense and resistant to breaking . . . each time there is a slight impact on a bone, as in running, a tiny piezo-electric current is generated," says Dr. J. Eschenberger, a research scientist working under the Association of Austrian Accident Insurance Companies. Remineralized bones are more osteoporosis-proof.

Exercise Plans for a Younger You

Like whole foods, whole body exercise can hold back the aging process if you give it half a chance. Which one's best to keep your body busy? That depends on what kind of shape you're in.

The first step is to have a head-to-foot physical that includes testing of both bones and muscles. Your physician should test the flexibility and strength of the legs, examine the hips and knees to determine their range of motion.

For example, if you sit on your haunches and one buttock doesn't reach the heel, it could be a sign of degenerative cartilage or arthritic changes in the knee. If you can't squat without discomfort, you may need flexibility drills. And if you've been sedentary, you may need to reverse the usual order of exercises used for younger people. Instead of aerobic exercises, such as swimming or skipping rope, stretching exercises for muscle and skeleton—and then aerobic exercises. Walking is considered the best so-called "entry" or beginner's exercise.

The second way to check out the shape you're in is to try out these five tests designed by the National Fitness Foundation—

1. *Arm Hang*

(Goal: Hang from the bar as long as possible—in minutes and seconds.)

Age	18–29	30–39	40–49	50–59	60 & over
Excellent					
Female	1:31+	1:21+	1:11+	1:01+	:51+
Male	2:01+	1:51+	1:35+	1:21+	1:11+
Very Good					
Female	:46–1:30	:40–1:20	:30–1:10	:30–1:00	:21– :50
Male	1:00–2:00	:60–1:50	:45–1:35	:35–1:20	:30–1:10
Good					
Female	to :45	to :39	to :29	to :29	to :20
Male	to :59	to :49	to :44	to :34	to :29

2. *Sit and Reach*

(Goal: Reach forward as far as possible while sitting—measure from crotch to fingertips—inches you can reach.)

Age	18–29	30–39	40–49	50–59	60 & over
Excellent					
Female	23+	23+	22+	21+	21+
Male	22+	22+	21+	20+	20+
Very Good					
Female	17–22	17–22	15–21	14–20	14–20
Male	15–21	13–21	13–20	12–19	19–18
Good					
Female	to 16	to 16	to 14	to 13	to 13
Male	to 12	to 12	to 12	to 11	to 11

3. *Curl-Ups*

(Goal: Do as many correct curl-ups as possible in one minute—number of curl-ups)

Age	18–29	30–39	40–49	50–59	60 & over
Excellent					
Female	46+	41+	36+	31+	26+
Male	51+	46+	41+	36+	31+
Very Good					
Female	25–45	20–40	18–35	12–30	11–32
Male	30–50	22–45	21–40	18–35	15–30
Good					
Female	to 24	to 19	to 15	to 11	to 10
Male	to 29	to 21	to 20	to 17	to 14

4. *3-Minute Step Test*

(Goal: Step up and down on a 12″ high bench in rhythm with a metronome; measure your heart rate after the exercise and compare it with these standards—heartbeats per minute)

Age	18–29	30–39	40–49	50–59	60 & over
Excellent					
Female	to 79	to 83	to 87	to 91	to 94
Male	to 74	to 77	to 79	to 84	to 89
Very Good					
Female	80–100	64–115	88–118	92–123	95–127
Male	75–100	78–108	80–112	85–115	90–118
Good					
Female	111+	116+	119+	124+	128+
Male	101+	110+	113+	116+	119+

5. *Push-Ups*

(Goal: Do as many push-ups as possible in one minute—number of pushups)

Age	18–29	30–39	40–49	50–59	60 & over
Excellent					
Female	46+	41+	36+	31+	26+
Male	51+	46+	41+	36+	31+
Very Good					
Female	17–45	12–40	8–35	6–30	5–25
Male	26–50	22–45	19–40	15–35	10–30
Good					
Female	to 16	to 11	to 7	to 5	to 4
Male	to 24	to 21	to 18	to 14	to 9

Step three is to get moving now that you know why being a twinkle toes is a better way of beating the Biological Time Clock than being a Twinkie addict. Here are a few pointers that apply no matter what you decide to try:

• Pick a sport (or pick two) you want to do that's well-suited to your condition, build and age. If it doesn't work out, forget it and try something else.

• Don't forget warm-up and cool-down periods: warm-ups allow arteries to dilate to provide adequate blood supply to the heart. Cooldowns allow the heart rate and blood pressure to come down gradually, taking the strain off the heart.

• Keep your workout wits about you: 30 minutes a session is sufficient, too much more may lead to injuries, decreased flexibility and stress or boredom. Three or four times a week is better than seven for the same reason.

• To get more out of less—add hand-held weights. They tone and strengthen major muscle groups throughout the body, promote general aerobic efficiency and help you burn 30% to 100% more calories.

THE 13 ACTIVITIES THAT HELP YOU STAY YOUNG LONGER

• *Ice Skating and Roller Skating*
  • University Studies Indicate Being a Good Skate Can Keep Your Heart Young
  • Skate to Prevent Pounds and Wrinkles
  • Reduce the Risk of Arthritis
  • Are You Built to Skate? Take This Doctor-Approved Test
  • Pointers for the Beginning Skater
• *Jumping Rope/Climbing Stairs/Stepping*
  • Why the American Medical Association Recommends Rope Jumping to Reverse the Aging Process
  • Skip More and Speed Weight Loss
  • Rope Jumping vs. Other Activities: What the Aerobics Research Institute Says
  • Skip Away Stress in 15 Minutes a Day
  • Is Skipping Rope an Aspirin Alternative?
  • 10-Week Program to Get the Jump on Aging
  • Burn the Calories in a Banana Split—Climb Stairs Daily
• *Walking*
  • Do You Know the Number One Reason Everyone Should Walk?
  • What Walking Does to Prevent Senility
  • Walking Makes Your Diet Work Better and Faster
  • Walk and You Can Throw Away Drugs and Pills
  • A Six-Month Program That Reduces the Risk of Heart Disease
  • Prevent Kidney Disease, Forgetfulness and Tired Blood with a Daily Stroll
  • Tips on Getting the Most Longevity Benefits out of Walking
• *Calisthenics*
  • Try the Lazy Bones Way to a Longer, Fitter Life
  • Seven Stay Young Benefits
  • Why Medical Experts Recommend Calisthenics to Improve Cardiovascular Health

- What Calisthenics Do for Life-Extension That Running and Cycling Don't
- Take Five Minutes a Day to Reverse Aging
- The One-to-One Fitness Center's 45-Minute Calisthenics Plan

- *Swimming*
  - Five Signs of Aging You Can Swim Away
  - Why the American College of Sports Medicine Calls Swimming a Top Age-Proofer
  - Swim to Boost Live-Longer Adrenalin Reserves
  - Five Ways Swimming Improves Your Lung Power
  - What an Easy Pool Workout Does for Your Heart
  - Easy Long-Life Pool Workout

- *Cycling*
  - Why Cycling Reduces Your Risk of Heart Disease
  - Burn the Calories in Two Banana Splits
  - Six Big Benefits of Cycling
  - Cycle to Improve Your Body's Longevity Vitamin D

- *Rebounding*
  - Mini-Jog Your Way to Super Health Without Leaving Home
  - Six Reasons Sports Physicians Rate Rebounding a Top Body Conditioner
  - How Rebounding Rejuvenates your Glands and Improves your Stress Tolerance
  - Rebounding, the Safest Sports Activity There Is
  - How to Get the Benefits of Running, Walking or Racquetball in 15 Minutes of Rebounding Daily

- *Parcours, the Swiss Total Body Workout*
  - Three Age-Proofing Benefits You Don't Get from Golf or Bowling
  - Get a Total Fitness Workout Without Leaving Home
  - Look Younger and Feel it in 30 Minutes a Day

- *Running/Jogging*
  - Why the Aerobic Institute Recommends Running at Any Age to Fight Aging
  - Look Like a 20-Year-Old at 70

- Best All-Around Cardiovascular-Conditioner, Says the Human Performance Laboratory
- Benefits of Running-in-Place
- Three-Week Rejuvenation Program
- *Racquet Sports—Tennis, Handball, Racquetball, Squash*
  - Why Racquet Sports Rate Tops as Whole Body Enhancers
  - The President's Council on Physical Fitness Calls Racquet Sports Good Fat-Fighters
  - How Courting Fitness Can Improve Your Diet
  - Why the Aerobic Institute Calls Racquet Sports "The Best Fitness in America"
  - Good Anti-Arthritis Activity
- *Weight Training*
  - The Easy Exercise That Could Increase Your Strength 20 to 30% in Two Weeks
  - Weight Training Protects You from Heart Disease, Says the AMA
  - Special Ways Women Benefit
  - More Get-Up-and-Go than You Get from Jogging or Cycling
  - Look Thinner in Eight Weeks
  - How to Reduce Your Body's Three Hot Spots for Fat
- *Martial Arts/Fencing*
  - The One Sport That Improves Your Mind as Well as Your Body
  - Why Martial Arts Produce Fitness Plus Tranquility
  - Burn as Many Calories as Jumping Rope
  - What You Get from Fencing That Boosts Youthful Vigor
  - Improve Your Brain-Power and Coordination
- *Yoga*
  - Would You Like to Know the Centuries Old Secret of Life-Long Flexibility?
  - Four Benefits of Yoga That Slow Aging
  - Yoga Provides a Key to Stress-Control and New Energy
  - An Anti-Arthritis Workout You Can Do in the Tub
  - End Lower Back Pain with These Two Exercises
  - Feel Better in 10 Ways with This One Exercise

University Studies Indicate Being a Good Skater Can Keep Your Heart Young

The baseball great Satchel Paige was once asked "How old would you *think* you were if you didn't *know* how old you were?" His answer was, "ageless." If yours isn't, consider rolling your way to rejuvenation.

What, skate when you could bowl? One reason—some sports do a better job than others in improving your physical fitness and in helping you avoid a heart attack which each year kills 600,000 mature Americans. And skating—on ice or wheels—is one of them. According to Dr. A. J. Selner of the University of California at Los Angeles, who studied the effects of skating five hours a week for 10 weeks, using women and men, 20 to 53, all previously sedentary non-skaters, there was an average 23% increase in leg strength, a decrease in cholesterol and triglyceride blood levels, a 9% improvement in protective HDL's (high density lipoproteins) in the blood and a 13% improvement in blood pressure.

Skate to Prevent Pounds and Wrinkles

Skating's a good match for swimming and tennis in terms of calorie burnoff (a 10 mph pace uses up 10 calories a minute, the equivalent of jogging at 5 mph or cycling at 10).

Skating's even aerobic enough to reverse wrinkles. According to Dr. James White, exercise physiologist and coordinator of physical fitness at the University of California, San Diego, studies of middle-aged athletes show that physical training affects the properties of the skin. The elastic quality that allows skin to spring right back to its original shape after being stretched is significantly better in the skin of athletes. People who exercise regularly, says White, "have fewer wrinkles than those who do not."[2] No wonder 60% of America's 50 million skaters are matrons not men.

Reduce the Risk of Arthritis

Being a good skater builds strength and flexibility if that's what your physical self is getting physical for. Skating also ranks as a good get-fit-and-make-friends activity. All you need is a sense of fun and a skate key and a nearby rink, and even that's not a must if you have an asphalt driveway outside.

Are you Built to Skate? Take This Doctor-Approved Test

On the other hand, it helps if you were born for wheeling and dealing. The key to that, according to Dr. Robert Arnot, director of the Sports Medicine Center at Lake Placid, New York and a physician for the U. S.

---

[2]To better that advantage, protect your skin from the aging effects of sunlight by wearing a sunscreen year long, advises the National Cancer Institute.

Olympic Ski Team and Winter Olympics, is that you have agility, endurance and a high vertical jump. These are the same traits that make skiing, tennis and gymnastics a piece of cake for a would-be fit 40-year-old.

If you fail the following test, consider running, walking or swimming: To test your vertical jump potential, stand next to a wall. Keeping feet flat, reach up as high as you can. Have a friend mark the wall at the tips of your fingers. Then, keeping your arm straight overhead, jump as high as you can. Mark this spot, too. Now measure the distance between the two marks. If it's 28 inches or more, you have an excellent jump; 22 to 28 inches is above average; 18 to 22 inches, average.

Pointers for the Beginning Skater

A few pointers before you start—

• Buy new skates that fit (a half or full size larger than shoe size). Don't start out with second-hand skates.

• Consider leather. It fits and wears better than synthetic.

• Have a pro check your heel attachments regularly to prevent lower leg and ankle fatigue.[3]

• To get all of the benefits of skating, aim for three sessions a week, 30–45 minutes a session. Or skate twice and substitute another activity such as brisk walking on exercise day three.

Longevity Benefits: *1, 3, 4, 5, 6, 8.*

JUMPING ROPE/CLIMBING STAIRS/STEPPING

Why the American Medical Association Recommends Rope-Jumping to Reverse the Aging Process

"There is no drug in current or prospective use that holds as much promise for sustained health as a lifetime program of physical exercise," says sports physician W. W. Bortz II in the *Journal of the American Medical Association* of 1982. What's Bortz's idea of a good low-cost aerobic exercise for getting a jump on aging? Jumping rope. It's not only good and ancient,[4] it's good and aerobic.

---

[3] If you *do* hurt after a healthy workout—what's healthier than aspirin? Head-to-toe massage. Call the American Massage and Therapy Association, Kingsport, Tennessee at (615)245-8071 for the massage pro nearest you. And if your hurt's an injury and there's nobody home but you—get professional advice by dialing a sports doctor at (317)926-1339. The 24-hour hotline is maintained by the University of Indiana School of Medicine.

[4] Nobody knows where rope skipping started, but jungle explorers in the last century returned from expeditions with tales of aborigines joyously jumping over vines and flexible strips of bamboo and pictures of medieval life shows tiny tots rolling hoops and jumping ropes.

Skip More and Speed Weight Loss

The burnoff is 720 calories an hour (at 120–140 turns per minute)—the same as running at a 5.7 mph pace—making it twice the calorie-busting workout of volleyball or table tennis. In fact, if you skip rope rather than skipping the first meal of the day to diet, 90% of what you lose will be dispensable fat, not indispensable, lean muscle, says cardiovascular expert Leonard Schwartz. "If you exercise 1,500 calories worth a day (this is five times the daily amount prescribed for fitness by the American Heart Association), you'll lose weight enormously fast." There's nothing to beat being on the ropes even if calorie burnoff's not your goal.

Rope Jumping vs. Other Activities: What the Aerobics Research Institute Says

Jumping rope, says Dr. Kenneth Cooper, founder of the Institute for Aerobics Research in Dallas, Texas, and inventor of the famous point system which measures the effectiveness of various kinds of exercise, doesn't take a back seat to any sport. Here's how it compares to a few of America's other popular ways of beating premature old age—

Activity	Time	Point Value (maximum points: 10)
Jumping rope	10 minutes	3 points
Jogging, 1 mile	10 minutes	3 points
Tennis, singles	1 30-minute set	1½ points
Swimming, 300 yards	10 minutes	1 point
Bicycling, 2 miles	8 to 10 minutes	1 point
Handball	10 minutes	1½ points
Walking, strolling	1 hour	1½ points

Skip Away Stress in 15 Minutes a Day

Skipping rope reduces tension, raises energy levels and works like a charm to produce total post-30 fitness fast. When participants in experiments at Illinois University's Physical Fitness Research Center were given ropes and asked to do as many turns as possible in five successive efforts and to do as many skips as possible in 60 minutes for five days each week for 10 weeks, the results were astonishing. Physical changes included greater leg and knee strength, increased calf size, better jumping ability (some could jump 4½ inches higher) and faster running speed. They were more agile, more flexible and their chests had deepened. Their hearts, instead of being strained, had become "vastly stronger."

Is Skipping Rope an Aspirin Alternative?

Skipping could even be an aspirin alternative. Why? Because exercising vigorously produces a high level of a natural opiate called beta-endorphin in response to strenuous activity, says Dr. Lee S. Berk, preventative medicine specialist in California's Loma Linda University. "This hormone-like substance produced by the brain and the pituitary gland increases the tolerance for pain and creates a feeling of well-being . . . The physically fit produce beta-endorphin more rapidly and in greater amounts than those who aren't."

10-Week Program to Get the Jump on Aging

Last but not least, anywhere you go, your rope can go with you. Here's an action plan to get the jump on aging. Don't leave home or end your day without it—

• *Before you begin*: Shop for a good rope—one of rawhide or one with plastic spaces over clothesline or ones covered with black sponge rubber. It should be just heavy enough to give you a good feel. (Even better, be a sport and invest $10 to $20 in the scientifically designed ropes all sport shops carry. Some even compute the twirls.)

• Hold the rope and stand with your feet on the middle. If the length is right, the handles will just reach your armpits.

• Use a jumping surface that's firm but cushioned: a low-pile carpet, or a cushy carpet remnant. Any hard surface is out; so are bare feet. Wear a good athletic shoe to prevent ankle and leg injuries.

• Warm up with a five-minute walk, then a slow stretching of the ankles, calves, shins and upper legs. Then follow the 15-week training schedule below. If you're a beginner, start at the top; if you're farther along, skip down the list to a more advanced stage. In either case, aim for 80 to 100 jumps per minute or 500 successive rope turns without missing in five minutes. Benefits of a skipping program begin to show up within a week.

• Alternate exercise and rest periods over the 15-week period and wear ankle or wrist weights to maximize cardiovascular benefits and increase calorie burnoff.

Week	Jump	Rest	Repeat	Total Jump Time
1	15 seconds	45 seconds	8 times	2 minutes
3	15 seconds	15 seconds	12 times	3 minutes
5	30 seconds	15 seconds	8 times	4 minutes
7	1 minute	30 seconds	7 times	7 minutes
9	2 minutes	1 minute	5 times	10 minutes
11	3 minutes	1 minute	5 times	15 minutes

Week	Jump	Rest	Repeat	Total Jump Time
13	6 minutes	1 minute	3 times	18 minutes
15	8 minutes	2 minutes	3 times	24 minutes

Burn the Calories in a Banana Split—Climb Stairs Daily

What else can touch jumping rope as a live-longer activity? Climbing stairs wherever you find them isn't bad, and neither is stepping. This activity can be done any time you have the urge and a standard 7-inch step or stool available. The procedure is to step onto the step and then down. A good rate is 25 up-and-down steps/minute while facing the same direction. Both burn about 7.5 calories per minute. (Twelve minutes of that kind of thing burns the calories in a baked potato—make it 79 and you can have a guilt-free banana split.) Best of all, it's aerobic.

Longevity Benefits: *1, 2, 3, 5, 7, 9.*

WALKING

If it's too late to become the baseball player you were meant to be, count your post-40 blessings. Being a Bingo Long has its bad points. According to Dr. Allan Ryan, M.D., editor of *Postgraduate Medicine and The Physician and Sportsmedicine*, "Baseball is not as good a cardiovascular conditioner as other fast sports, the chances for incurring injury are high and you don't play baseball to *get* fit, you must *be* fit to play it."

Do You Know the Number-One Reason Everyone Should Walk?

Walking is the least demanding and probably the most rewarding of all the indoor/outdoor activities you can do after 40, and it may be the *only* one you can *keep* doing. Thirty-eight percent of all U.S. 50- to 59-year-olds walk for fitness, and walking is one of the chief reasons so many of Pakistan's Hunzas live to be 100-plus, says Dr. Roy Walford of UCLA. In addition to their healthy apricot-chili-pepper-and-glacial-water diet, they walk daily up and down 500-foot hills.

When a patient of former White House physician, Dr. Paul Dudley White, came in for a checkup at age 102, for example, he was advised to continue walking his customary mile a day. He lived to be 107. An Arab named Touat Mohand Said walked 93 miles to Algiers at the age of 109 to claim his pension.

What Walking Does to Prevent Senility

Walking might be the best way to prevent senility as well. According to results of a four-month program of brisk walking initiated at the University of Utah, exercise builds mental "muscles" and may postpone aging's effects on the brain. (Aerobic exercise makes the body better at transporting oxygen to all your organs, your brain included.) Researchers said all of the study's participants were better able to remember sequences of numbers and use abstract thinking to correctly match numbers and symbols at the conclusion of the walking program.

Walking keeps you slim and trim without pain. The American Medical Association recommends you get at least 300 calories of exercise a day after 40. An hour of strutting your stuff at a brisk 120-steps-a-minute-pace-with-purpose fills the bill. In addition, says Dr. Kenneth Cooper, director of the Aerobics Institute in Dallas, "A pace of 5 miles an hour for 45 minutes exercises the cardiovascular system as effectively as 30 minutes of moderate aerobic dancing—and burns the same number of calories. Walking 3 miles in an hour helps you develop good muscle tone and it metabolizes a lot of fat."

Walking Makes Your Diet Work Better and Faster

If you're already walking, in fact, adding 1 mile a day beyond your quota even *without* a change in diet, should result in the loss of a pound every 36 days, and save on chiropractor/podiatrist calls. "Unlike jogging—which has a very high injury rate—walking poses almost no hazard at all," states Dr. Bob Karch, executive director of the National Center for Health Fitness in Washington, D.C. Just make sure you strut your stuff wearing good shoes—that means a raised heel, a padded insole and a fabric that breathes (a canvas and leather combination is good). Add socks of hi-bulk orlon or rayon and you're in business.

Walk and You Can Throw Away Drugs and Pills

Simple as it seems, walking actually involves the synchronization of many of the body's more than 200 bones, over 650 muscles and some 70,000 miles of circulatory channels. And it's worth the stay-young effort. According to researchers at the University of Massachusetts Center for Health, Fitness and Human Performance, "The physiological benefits of walking are enormous . . . Circulating blood, with its oxygen and vital nutrients, from head to toe is no small task. The hard part is getting all those corpuscles back to the heart. Expanding and contracting foot muscles, calves, thighs and buttocks help pump the blood back. Circulatory sluggishness due to lack of exercise increases the heart's work, with a resulting increase in heart rate and blood pressure, and a higher risk of disease."

A Six-Month Program That Reduces the Risk of Heart Disease

In fact, says Dr. James Rippe, director of the University of Massachusetts Center for Health, Fitness and Human Performance, do your paces for six months and you may never need a pacemaker. "Aerobic capacity virtually increases by 15 to 20%—that's 30% above the average American."

But that's not all!

Prevent Kidney Disease, Forgetfulness and Tired Blood with a Daily Stroll

The aging kidneys also get a hand from your moving feet. An acupuncture point located just behind the ankle bone relates to kidney acid which can cause a toxic condition in the blood and contribute to sluggishness of mind and body. "The rhythmic motion and increased oxygenation of the brain that occurs in walking are conducive to relaxation and even creative problem solving . . . Action absorbs anxiety," says stress authority Dr. Hans Selye.

What else do you need to know to get the most out of the world's least complicated sport? Here are some tips once you lace up.

Tips on Getting the Most Long-Life Benefits out of Walking

• Practice good posture when walking for a more efficient stride. Keep your head high and your back erect, and tuck in your buttocks.

• Your feet should be spaced 2 to 4 inches apart. Reach out with your hip, knee and heel, and point your toes in the direction of travel.

• Make the back edge of the heel strike first, with the ankle set only slightly to the outside.

• Let your arms swing naturally in an arc about the shoulder to increase speed, maintain rhythm and keep the upper body toned.

• A longer stride is the key to walking faster and burning more calories per step.

• And don't do your brisk beach walking in your bare feet. According to Dr. Adrian Lees of the Sports Biomechanics Department at Liverpool Polytechnic in England, exercising without shoes puts even greater pressure on your foot and flattens the way you land, causing you to stress muscles. Prolonged barefoot exercise can also lead to knee and ankle injuries, even knee and hip disorders.

An easy longevity program for older beginners—

1. Start with a 15-minute walk every other day for two weeks; increase to 30 minutes over the next two weeks. Gradually work up to four 45- to 60-minute sessions a week.

2. Pace isn't important, just be comfortable. Two miles an hour (slow) or 3 miles (moderate) is acceptable. Four miles an hour (fast) may be too demanding.

3. Strive for regularity and consistency. If it's easier to walk for a half hour *every* day rather than an hour every *other* day, do it. Fifteen minutes morning and evening and 30 minutes at lunchtime bring the same results as a continuous one-hour walk, too. But for best aerobic (heart-lung) benefits, no session should be *shorter* than 15 minutes. A good goal if you're feeling good is an average of 3 miles a day, 5 days a week at a pace of 5 miles an hour.

Longevity Benefits: *1, 2, 3, 7, 8, 9.*

CALISTHENICS

Try the Lazy Bones Way to a Longer, Fitter Life

Calisthenics is a good lazy bones way to lengthen your time on the planet even if taking things sitting and lying down doesn't look like much. The trick is deciding on *which* lazy, easy thing to do and how long and how often to do it.

Seven Long-Life Benefits

Calisthenics[5] do more to increase body strength than improve cardiovascular and respiratory stamina, which is why they make a good prelude for a better-ranked workout such as running. On the other hand, you do burn more calories than bowling, the injury risk is low, you don't have to do it outdoors and, like other push-and-pull activities, calisthenics helps you fight off calcium and circulatory disorders such as osteoporosis and varicose veins.

Why Medical Experts Recommend Calisthenics to Improve Cardiovascular Health

According to Brointo Kiveloff, M.D., associate chief of Rehabilitation Medicine at the New York infirmary-Beekman Downtown Hospital, a sound cardiovascular system needs good reserves of blood properly distributed through the body. Normally, the muscles store some 40 to 50% of the body's total blood supply—and aging affects blood-storing muscle fiber, replacing it with connective tissue which can't store blood nearly as well. Isometric exercises attack these problems by improving circulation, muscle tone and bulk and lowering blood pressure; they even prevent wrinkles and improve posture.

---

[5]Calisthenics cover both isometrics and isotonics. (In the first you flex muscles without moving them, the second invovles pullup-pushup movement.)

What Calisthenics Do for Living Longer That Running and Cycling Don't

In fact, according to Dr. Phillip Felig of Yale University, the calisthenic arm exercises use more energy than leg-dependent activities, give you a more complete workout and are the reason orchestra conductors like Arturo Toscanini, for example, lived to the ripe old age of 90.

Take Five Minutes a Day to Reverse Aging

Here's a simple life-extending example of isometrics in action, and all it takes is five minutes a day—

1. Stand in a relaxed position, arms hanging loose. Don't clench your fists, but bend your elbows or other joints.
2. Tense all your muscles at the same time as tightly as possible, while breathing normally and counting aloud to six. You can try tensing each muscle group separately—legs, arms, chest, abdomen, face—and then try tensing them all at once. You should feel an immediate surge of warmth.
3. Relax and rest for a few seconds.
4. Repeat two more times and do three times a day.

The One-to-One Fitness Center's 45-Minute Calisthenics Plan

Better yet, here's a one-size-fits-all-longevity calisthenics plan to work into any live-longer life plan. Do the "six flab-busters" exercise plan below—include a little aerobic warm-up plus stretching and cool-down. Do it 45 minutes three times a week and you'll be fit for life, says the program director of the One-to-One Fitness Center in New York City. All you need is one 10-pound weight, one 5-pound weight, an exercise mat, a towel and a pair of running shoes. To get maximum benefits, do two sets of everything.

1. *Warmup.* Kick off your workout with aerobics—brisk walking or jogging. To reap heart/lung building and calorie-burning benefits, keep going for 20 to 30 minutes. Move in place to music, or take to the streets. Start with a warmup walk for five minutes. Then jog a few blocks, walk a few, jog a few, walk a few—until you can run the entire time. Within six weeks you should cover 2–3 miles. Cool down with a five-minute walk before doing strengthening exercises.
2. *Firm-up.* Stand about 2½ feet from a sturdy table (or bookcase or counter). Keeping back straight, lean forward and grasp tabletop. Bend left leg at the knee and raise foot behind you. Without twisting back, lift bent left leg to side, then slowly straighten leg. Hold for a count of two, bend knee and lower. Build up to 20. On the last lift, hold for 80 seconds. Reverse legs. Repeat.
3. *Leg-Shapers.* Lie on left side, resting on left elbow. Place right foot in front of left knee. Lift left leg as high as possible, then lower without

allowing leg to touch the ground. Build to 20, holding the last "lift" for 10 seconds. Repeat on right side.

4. *Scissors Kicks for Abdomen Strength*: Lie on back, fingers laced behind neck, elbows out. Raise head slightly, press lower back into mat at all times. Lift left leg straight up and raise right leg one foot. Then "scissor"— alternatively raising legs, dropping lower leg only to point that back is still flat to mat. Build to 20 each leg, holding last lift for each leg 10 seconds.

5. *Waist-Trimmer*. Lie on back with knees bent, legs slightly apart, arms at sides. Contract stomach and curl up halfway reaching to left of knees. Do 10. Repeat to right side. Then reach to center for 10 seconds. Add a second set when this is easy.

6. *Hamstring and Across-the-Chest Stretching*: Stand with feet shoulder's width apart, arms out to the sides. Reach right hand down and across body to outside of left calf, twisting torso and letting left knee bend slightly. Point left arm to ceiling. Feel stretch in straight leg and across back. Hold for 30 seconds, repeat with other leg. Then, stand with feet slightly apart, arms at sides. Hold one end of a bath-size towel in each hand. Raise arms straight up, over and behind you, and hold for 30 seconds.

Longevity Benefits: *3, 4, 5.*

SWIMMING

Five Signs of Aging You Can Swim Away

Time plays many tricks. There are eight you can't debate—hair grays, gets dry and thins; skin sags; teeth loosen; wrinkles appear; breasts sag; posture and flexibility diminish; age spots appear and flab becomes more apparent—to say nothing of added pounds. But out of eight, there are five[6] you can do something about, and swimming's one of the best ways to do it.

Why the American College of Sports Medicine Calls Swimming a Top Age-Proofer

According to the American College of Sports Medicine, running gets top marks as a heart-health activity and a waist-down conditioner, but for a workout that age-proofs the rest of you without the stress that running exerts on the joints, you're better off learning to love laps. (Only aerobic dancing and cross-country skiing get as many fitness brownie points.)

Swimming builds muscular endurance and strength as a result of the natural water resistance, exercises the shoulders and ankles more than any

---

[6]Keeping teeth intact, retarding wrinkles and age spots is something you have to leave to nutrition.

sport[7] with the possible exception of no-nonsense weight training and is the sport of choice if you are overweight, says Dr. Willibald Nagler, physiatrist-in-chief at the New York Hospital—Cornell Medical Center. All you need is a swimsuit and membership at the Y.

Swim to Boost Time-Fighting Adrenalin Reserves

Swimming also benefits the nervous system. Even a gentle workout increases the secretion of adrenalin, an anti-aging juice that helps regulate your whole basal metabolic rate. This establishes essential processes in your body that keep you looking and feeling like the young old-timer you were meant to be. Swimming improves muscle size and tone, firms flabby muscles, increases size of muscle fibers and produces an increased blood supply to the muscles permitting more nutrients to feed more muscle—and muscular endurance is also boosted.

Five Ways Swimming Improves Your Lung Power

What's more, swimming gives your respiratory system as good a run for the money as running. The rhythmic action of swimming helps improve the exchange of oxygen and carbon dioxide between body cells; it also increases the rate and depth of breathing so more oxygen is made available for fuel production and for the removal of carbon dioxide and other toxic wastes and irritants. Swimming enables you to breathe more efficiently and increases the size and capacity of the capillaries in the lungs so that more oxygen is absorbed.

What an Easy Pool Workout Does for Your Heart

Swimming meets the criteria of aerobics authorities as a sport that metabolizes fats from the bloodstream and qualifies for being an exercise that can be done at a relatively low intensity for a long period of time. This

---

[7]Do you need this benefit? You do if you fail the following test:

Test for Upper Torso/Stomach Strength

(Do as many pushups as possible in one minute)

Age	18–29	30–39	40–49	50–59	60 & over
Excellent					
Female	46+	41+	36+	31+	26+
Male	51+	46+	41+	36+	31+
Very Good					
Female	17–45	12–40	8–35	6–30	5–25
Male	26–50	22–45	19–40	15–35	10–30
Good					
Female	to 16	to 11	to 7	to 5	to 4
Male	to 24	to 21	to 18	to 14	to 9

means it is a way to prevent strokes.[8] Swimming improves the action of the heart, contracts thigh and leg muscles, and squeezes the veins, thus helping to pump blood back to your heart. The returning blood enables your heart to beat with more energy. This improves circulation and overall vitality.

Two final pluses—swimming gets top marks for sociability from the President's Council on Physical Fitness, and aerobics pioneer Dr. Kenneth Cooper, says, "There is a rhythmical sensation in swimming not dissimilar to that of dancing, and there is the pleasant feel of the water enveloping and soothing the entire body."

And last, but not least, if you really get in the swim of things, you burn 500 to 900 calories an hour.[9]

Easy Life-Extending Pool Workout

If you'd like to get thin, not just wet—here's an easy, in-pool time-fighter workout to use two or three times a week. (Any calisthenics you can comfortably do submerged, do.)

Do 20 repetitions of each exercise below and increase the number of repetitions or add waterproof ankle and wrist weights[10] as you improve. You will be amazed at how easy it is to shape up without even breaking into a sweat.

1. *Bobbing.* Use this as a warmup as well as a cool-down from your workout. Develops your ability to breathe deeply. Stand in the pool in water waist-deep or higher. Extend arms to the sides. Inhale deeply through nose and mouth. As you bend your knees, exhale completely, forming bubbles, and come up. Repeat this exercise at least 10 times, rest. Repeat.

2. *Pool Wall Push-Ups.* Strengthens your arms, the shoulders and the back of your legs. Face pool wall and rest palms on the edge, elbows bent, hands shoulder-width apart. Bend knees and jump up, straightening arms

---

[8]If you'd rather ride a stationary bike than ride the waves, it provides the same benefits as swimming, says the Institution of Sports Medicine at Lennox Hill Hospital.

[9]Here are 7 snack-happy rewards of a 7- to 32-minute swim:

To Burn Calories in	Food	Swim for (minutes)
101	apple, large	9
108	slice of bread and butter	7
356	cake, 1/12, two-layer type	32
166	milk, 8 oz glass	15
108	potato chips, 10	10
396	spaghetti & sauce, 1½ cups	5
350	hamburger	31

[10]Even better, invest in a strap-on "wet vest" which increases calorie burnoff and aerobic benefits invented by Glenn McWaters, president of the Sports Medicine and Fitness Institute in Birmingham, Alabama, and sold at sports apparel shops.

and lifting your body so that front of thighs rest on the edge. Tense your body and hold for five seconds, then ease your body back down into the water.

3. *Sit-Ups*. Strengthens abdomen and front of legs. With back to wall, grasp pool edge or gutter with arms fully extended to each side. Press legs together, bend and lift them up, tucking knees to chest. Extend legs straight out, tuck into chest, then lower; place feet on pool floor. Repeat. Try these in a floating position, holding a kick-board over abdomen for support.

4. *Kicking*. Strengthens legs and provides aerobic benefits. Done correctly, this helps improve your swimming kick. Hold onto the pool wall for support and practice the flutter kick, scissors kick, breaststroke whip kick or butterfly dolphin kick. Do each of the different kicking exercises first while floating on your stomach, then again while on your back.

Longevity Benefits: *1, 2, 3, 4, 5, 6, 8, 9*.

CYCLING

Why Cycling Reduces Your Risk of Heart Disease

According to Dr. Robert Brown, professor of psychology at the University of Virginia, the natural-born bicyclist is an idealist, enterprising and a self-starter. He's also getting all the live-longer benefits of running or swimming without doing either.

"Wise men who have bicycled vigorously for most of their lives are 10 times less likely to develop heart disease than are others their age," says Dr. H. K. Robertson, director of Great Britain's Fellowship of Cycling Old Timers. And health records of the club's 300 members indicate that cyclists have less heart disease and fewer heart attacks. Those over age 75 appeared to enjoy the greatest protection as a result of their lifelong exercise—10-fold.

According to the Aerobics Institute, the training affects and benefits the internal organs and is identical to the benefits of running and swimming—or better. It meets the criteria for a top-level, low-intensity exercise that builds strength, improves flexibility, helps metabolize fat rapidly in the body and improves cardiovascular fitness. But you can't make it easy on yourself. To earn those 20 aerobic points (that's 5 more than swimming), the effort must be continuous at an 8 to 13 mph speed.

Burn the Calories in Two Banana Splits

A cyclist who covers 20 miles an hour gets the workout equivalent of a 10-mile run. In terms of weight loss, cycling for one hour at a good clip burns the calories in one to two banana splits (300 to 600), making it calorie buster number three (after running and cross-country skiing).

Six Big Benefits of Cycling

Here's a rundown of some of biking's biggest benefits to get you started—

• Promotes a more efficient pumping of the blood from the extremities to the heart by the constant, rhythmic leg movement.

• Causes a big increase in the heart's volume and a slower heart rate—both factors in lowering blood pressure.

• Prompts improved blood flow to the brain, improving the tiger-in-your-tank potential.

• Reduces the possibility of a slipped disk through the strengthening of back muscles; also improves mood, emotional stability and general health. And it makes you sweat. Perspiration is an important stay-young factor because of a derangement of cell metabolism, caused mainly by the accumulation of waste products in the tissues, which interferes with the nourishment and oxygenation of the cells. It is estimated that one-third of all body impurities are excreted through the skin. More than a pound of waste is discharged every day. Your skin, in other words, is an organ of detoxification. Bettering its sweat potential by biking could help lengthen your life.

Cyle to Improve Your Body's Age-Proofing Vitamin D

And last, but not least, cycling may be the best antidote for stress and fatigue there is, says the League of American Wheelmen. It gets you outdoors for fresh air and a dose of vitamin D-rich, longer-life sunshine.

Cycling's one drawback? Because it isolates the thighs and most of your push power is supplied by hips and legs, the greatest strengthening effect goes to these areas.

And if cycling will never replace soap operas for you, make it easy on yourself. Bring America's favorite outdoor sport indoors. Just be sure to invest in a good one with tension levers that let you increase the pedaling burden plus a speedometer that tells you how fast you'd be moving if you were on the open road. (See *Health Gadgets*, page 221.)

What's the right routine once you've got the right bike at the right price? Thirty to 45 minutes of freewheeling three times a week will do it.

Longevity Benefits: *1, 2, 3, 4, 7.*

REBOUNDING

Mini-Jog Your Way to Super Health Without Leaving Home

Regret that you're not a runner? Count your athletic blessings. "Too much running on hard surfaces actually destroys red blood cells in the body," says *The Physician and Sports Medical Journal*, explaining why runners and other endurance athletes are so susceptible to development of low red blood cell counts and other signs of "sports anemia."

Six Reasons Sports Physicians Rate Rebounding a Top Body Conditioner

What *can* you do if you want to take your exercise but take it easy? Buy a rebounder. Getting in your aerobic ups and downs on a mini-trampoline may possibly be the best all-around body conditioner around. According to exercise physiologist Charles Kuntzleman, Ed.D., it can help improve your body symmetry, improve flexibility, help build muscle, bulk and strength and it's kidstuff.

Rebounding beats a full evening of bowling all hollow as a sweat-debt sport. Three games on the lanes gives you only three minutes of *real* cardiovascular exercise, says the Director of the President's Council on Physical Fitness and Sports. Ditto other easy-going workouts like golf, a very low intensity sport that does near-zero for aerobic fitness—softball, for instance, actually occupies second to last place on the Council Maximum Benefit Sports Scoreboard, it burns only 750 calories an hour (three times as many as a single household chore like window cleaning or vacuuming).

Rebounding is done on a rebounder—a disc-shaped canvas- and/or net-covered platform that resembles a miniature trampoline (also called mini-joggers, skip-joggers, globe-joggers). The basic structure and function of the apparatus is generally the same though they may vary in appearance. Rebounding offers the benefits of jogging without the drawbacks, and unlike running, which puts a gravity pull of 2.7 on your body, rebounding reduces gravity's pull to 1.05—just a little more than if you were standing but with the cardiovascular effects of vigorous movement. And the more you reduce gravity's pull, the more you minimize the effects of the aging process which could eliminate sagging jowls and a double chin.

How does rebounding measure up compared to other fitness activities? Twenty minutes of up-and-down exercise is equal to jogging 3½ miles in 32 minutes; 40 minutes of handball or racquetball; 15 minutes of jumping rope (110 steps per minute) or 2½ miles of walking in 34 minutes, says Dr. Morton Walker, a specialist in preventive medicine. Rebounding also increases lung capacity and reduces heart attack risk, adds the Stamford, Connecticut physician who also feels it reduces cancer risk by super-oxygenating cells—all 60 trillion—through the force of gravity. "At the bottom of a bounce, you're at double gravity. The double pressure pushes waste products from cells at twice the normal rate. At the top, you're at zero gravity. Cells take in twice the amount of oxygen."

How Rebounding Rejuvenates Your Glands and Improves Your Stress Tolerance

Done long enough and vigorously enough, rebounding increases the body's reserve of beta-endorphin, a hormone which the brain and the pituitary gland produce to increase pain tolerance, counteract stress and impart a feeling of well-being.

Rebounding, The Safest Sports Activity There Is

Other bonuses? Rebounding's non-competitive, doesn't require lessons, can be started at any age, has the lowest injury potential of all sports this side of swimming or walking and it doesn't expose you to choking auto exhaust or snarling dogs. And if you get a portable trampoline, you never have to leave home without it. The initial investment, slightly over $100 including a book and maybe an audio cassette of routines, is no more than a year's membership at the YMCA, and it's a gift to yourself that keeps giving. You can get it at any well-stocked sporting goods shop.

How to Get the Benefits of Running, Walking or Racquetball in 15 Minutes of Rebounding Daily

Once you've got it? Here's how to use it—

• Before you start, stretch properly, then spring up and down gently just to get the feel of this "mini"-trampoline. Test out your balance. Walk by easily lifting one leg up and then the other. Quicken the pace by swinging your arms slightly.

• After you get accustomed to the active sway and bounce of the tramp, you can increase your rebound adding new exercises as you go. For example:

1. *The Rebound Runner*: Stand in the center of the tramp. Start a leisurely walk, jog or running motion. Lift knees as high as you can. Without waiting for the rebounder to bounce back, pick up speed. Keep going three minutes or more. Rest and repeat. (*Note*: The faster the motion and the higher the knees rise, the greater the aerobic benefit.)

2. *The Tramp Twist*: Start in the middle of the tramp. Bounce so that while your hips and legs turn to the left, your chest and shoulders twist to the right. On the second bounce, turn the hips and legs to the right and the chest and shoulders to the left. Repeat once in each direction. Rest. Repeat. (*Note*: To get the most benefits, work hard and don't rest too long. When you stop, calorie burnoff drops off as much as 30 to 50%.)

Like to net a bigger net gain? Find out how many ups and downs equal a piece of cake by wearing a calorie-computed clipper to your belt. Two which sell for less than $100 that catch every last incoming, outgoing calorie are *Cal Count* and *Cal Trak*.

Longevity Benefits: *2, 3, 4, 5, 6.*

PARCOURS, THE SWISS TOTAL BODY WORKOUT

Three Stay-Young Benefits You Don't Get from Golf or Bowling

Is golf or bowling your chosen workout? You could have picked better: on a scale of 1 to 10, the lanes and tees may have "just sitting on your hands" beat aerobically, but not by much. Both golf and bowling rate a "10" for competition from the Aerobic Institute, but near-zero for their conditioning, strengthening, figure-shaping and life-lengthening benefits.

There's a better way to put fun and fitness in your life. Try an indoor or outdoor parcours. It consists of a series of intelligently planned, on-the-spot exercises that are interspersed with spurts of running, jogging or walking, performed on a prearranged route. Parcours was developed by a Swiss insurance company in Zurich concerned about improving the fitness level of its employees. The idea caught on. Today, there are hundreds of courses throughout Switzerland, Germany and Sweden. In fact, Zurich's better-idea-for-better-bodies has exercise enthusiasts everywhere "making the rounds."

Get a Total Fitness Workout Without Leaving Home

Parcours popularity is no surprise. Completing all the given exercises at each "station" gives you a total fitness workout that benefits your heart, lungs and every one of the body's muscle groups—the ones at your waist not excluded.[11] You don't need to get out your bike, buy special gear or (if you've got the indoor variety) wait for good weather. According to the President's Council on Physical Fitness, parcours will improve your breathing, make your circulation more efficient and improve your posture. And if you like being a lonely-only exerciser, parcours is for you, since you can do it without a partner.

---

[11]If you feel like you've lost fat at the middle, maybe you have. A good gadget that will tell you is a Skinfold Caliper which determines total amount of fat on your body, computes your true ideal weight and monitors any change in muscle tissue when dieting or exercising. At sporting good stores for about $20, or write Creative Health Products, 410 Saddleridge Road, Plymouth, Michigan 48170.

Look Younger and Feel It in 30 Minutes a Day

Calorie burnoff? That depends on how long and how vigorously you work out, and also how much you weigh (the more you weigh, the more calories you use). Thirty minutes at a moderate pace is good for a minimum of 200–300 calories if you weigh 120 pounds. That makes parcours the caloric equivalent of jazz dancing or bicycling. And just adding wrist, ankle or handheld weights will up the thin-down effect by 30%.

Indoor parcours

• Choose five stations throughout the house—areas next to your dining room table, your bedroom dresser, study desk, kitchen counter and livingroom couch, for example.

• Write instructions (below) on a sheet of paper. At station #1, post a sheet of paper with the instructions for the stretching exercises. At #2, instructions for jumping jacks, etc. Wear comfortable exercise clothes and sneakers.

Outdoor parcours

• If you're using your yard, plan on a 6-foot-wide track, 2½ miles long. At intervals along the track set up 10 to 20 stations to which you can walk or jog, according to the posted directions.

• At each station do a different set of exercises, starting with a simple warmup and progressing to harder exercises, then a wind-down and cool-down activity.

Now—here's how it's actually done:

Parcours instructions

Warm-up by walking a brisk two minutes.

Station #1: Stretching

Stand one arm's length from the wall, palms flat against it. Bending your elbows and supporting your body's weight on your hands, lean forward until your forehead touches the wall. Keep heels on the ground; push upright again. Repeat three times.

From an erect standing position, lunge forward onto your right foot, keeping your left heel flat. Bend right knee deeper to feel a stretch in your thighs. Lunge forward onto left foot.

Jog in place five minutes.

Station #2: Jumping Jacks

Do 10 with big broad movement for a good workout.

Station #3: Windmills

Do 10, raise arms to your sides at shoulder level, twisting around to the right from the waist. After twisting to the right, twist to the left. Repeat nine more times.

Jog in place five minutes.

Station #4: Knee-touches

Do three. Sit on the floor with legs spread out to either side. Lean forward over your right leg and touch knee with your outstretched hands. Lean farther forward and touch toes with hands. Repeat.

Jump rope for two minutes.

Station #5: Leg stretch

Place leg on a waist-high piece of furniture. Lean forward over leg and s-t-r-e-t-c-h. Repeat with opposite leg, then lie on floor with feet tucked under a sofa. Knees should be slightly bent to protect the back. Hands behind your head. Roll up into a sitting position, then roll back down to the floor. Repeat 10 times.

Cool-down by walking; shaking out your arms and hands at your sides and rotating your head as you go. Tired and tingling? If you feel 10 years younger, you've done everything right.

Ready for more? To get more details on parcours and a more ambitious self-help program, write the American Alliance for Health, Physical Education and Recreation, 1201 16th Street N.W., Washington, D.C. 20036.

Longevity Benefits: *1, 2, 3, 5, 7.*

RUNNING/JOGGING

Why the Aerobic Institute Recommends Running at Any Age to Fight Aging

If you've mastered walking and you're hot to trot, don't let age or sex stand in the way. "What I like most about running," says The Aerobics Institute director Dr. Kenneth Cooper, "is that I can recommend it to anyone of any age." Amos Alonzo Stagg, the former famous University of Chicago football coach, played tennis until age 83, then switched to running. He continued to jog in his backyard until age 96, when the cataracts in his eyes became so bad he began bumping into trees.

Make Your Body Look Like a 20-Year-Old's at 70

Running or jogging,[12] in fact, may be the best exercise of all to prevent that 10% per-decade decline in physical fitness that goes with getting older, according to Dr. Michael Pollock of the University of Wisconsin Mount Sinai Medical Center. In a fitness study that Pollack directed, the aerobic capacity (VO_{max}) of 25 30-plus runners were tested, then retested after a lapse of 10 years to see what shape they were in. Results? Those who were still running showed no fall-off in aerobic capacity; while those who reduced training showed a slight decline, but were still in the top percentile for their age group. "If you put bags over their heads, you'd think they were 20-year-olds . . (yet) some of these men were in their 70's," says Pollock.

A lot of America's older road runners are women these days, too. In 1972, the New York City L'eggs Mini Marathon for women drew 78 entrants; in 1985 5,690 came. Today, there are roughly 7 million women runners in the U.S. and 5% of them doing roadwork are well past their prime.

True, running's not every man or woman's beat-the-biological-time-clock sport. "Running can strain the joints, particularly if done on hard roads or in poorly fitting shoes. Knees, ankles and achilles tendons often suffer and sprinting (all-out running) can produce muscle tears," warns the American College of Sports Medicine. Running's also too taxing if you're a good-and-plenty prime-of-lifer (swimming's a better bet if you're a bit overweight). Running's too weight-reductive if you're already too thin, also. After six months to a year of faithful running, women often find that their bra size has shrunk along with their waistline.

Running, like swimming and hiking, is best suited to individuals with excellent endurance and only middling agility. Golf, bowling or sailing, advises the Olympic Sports Medicine Center at Lake Placid, New York, are the sports to consider if you have poor endurance and excellent agility.

Best All-Around Cardiovascular Conditioner, Says the Human Performance Laboratory

On the plus side—running ranks as the most efficient of all the live-longer activities. Runners have denser bones than the golfers and the differences have been shown to be directly related to the stress running

---

[12]For practical considerations, running and jogging are the same activity; jogging is simply slow running. The difference between runners and joggers is mostly state of mind.

puts on limbs, say researchers at the Mayo Clinic and National Health Systems in Ann Arbor, Michigan. And you earn five fat aerobic points in just eight fast minutes (if you go for them with golf, it will take you 7 hours).

Losing weight? No other activity comes close to footwork with the exception of rowing or scull racing. According to sports Dr. Robert J. Johnson of the University of Illinois, running at 10 miles per hour can burn up to 900 calories (90 calories per mile). Even jogging along at an easy 12 minutes per mile pace burns 450 calories every 60 minutes.

Running benefits every muscle group in the body, tones arm muscles and flattens the stomach. But its most important benefit is cardiovascular (heart/lungs), the one most of us need the most. According to physiologist David L. Costill of the Human Performance Laboratory at Ball State University, "In order to metabolize excessive fats from your blood stream, you need to exercise at relatively low intensity and for long periods. That's why nothing can equal running for benefitting your heart."

Benefits of Running-in-Place

And what could be simpler? You can run or jog anywhere in any weather. All you need are thick-soled shoes made just for running, walking or hiking (sneaker-wearing can lead to disabling foot problems) and a good pair of high-bulk orlon or other synthetic fabric sweat socks.

And what if you are a swimmer first? Become a runner on your non-pool days. A good jog is a fun way to meet your exercise quota and beat exercise boredom.

Runner's guide to fluid replacement

The weight you lose after a run is a better guide than thirst to how much fluid you need to drink during your exercise day. Count on one pint of fluid for every 3 pounds lost. Water's best, but if you want something tastier here's how to mix it for the best energy effect, says the ACSM:

Drink	Calories/8 oz.	Carbohydrate g./8 oz.	Parts Water to Add
Energade	120	30	5
Gatorade	48	12	2
Apple juice	120	29.6	5
Orange juice	122	28.9	5
V-8 juice	47	10.6	2
Seven-up	96	24	4

Starter Program for Runners/Joggers

Can't wait to be off and running? Here are four final tips and a program to follow:

• Don't forget warm-up and cool-down periods: a 10-minute warmup causes arteries to dilate, ensuring an adequate blood supply to the heart. Cool-downs allow the heart rate and blood pressure to come down gradually, taking the strain off your heart.

• Keep your workout wits about you. A 30-minute run/jog is enough, more can lead to injuries, loss of flexibility and stress or boredom. And three to four times a week is better than seven for the same reason.

• To get more out of less, tote weights—the right ones. Weights improve muscle tone and increase calorie burnoff by 30%, according to Bryant Stamford, Ph.D., director of the Exercise Physiology Laboratory, University of Louisville School of Medicine. "It's the extra upper-body work that increases calorie/fat burnoff." Start with 1 pound and add in 1-pound increments. Pick handheld weights that loop or strap on to avoid the gripping which can cause muscle fatigue. Ankle weights raise your injury risk, says Stamford.

• As for gear? The tight stuff is the right stuff. Look for the new lycra and nylon body-tights. They fit like a second skin and keep you warm for $40 or less.

Three-Week Rejuvenation Program

	Level	Goal (Distance (either)	(or)	Frequency
Week One Week	Walk continuously at a comfortable pace Walk/run	30 minutes	30 minutes	4 times a week
Two	Run at least twice during the period but don't strain	1 mile	30 minutes	4 times a week
Week Three	Run/walk Aim for a routine that involves running and walking equally	1½ miles	25 minutes	4 times a week

• *Your goal*: A mile, or 10 to 12 minutes of running.

• Like to check out a few more running programs? Write International Running and Fitness Association, 2420 K Street, N.W., Washington, D.C. 20037.

• Accident prone? Protect yourself with a copy of "Playing It Safe! A Pocket Guide to Fitness" from the National Safety Council, PR Dept., 444 No. Michigan Avenue, Chicago, IL 60611

Longevity Benefits: *1, 2, 3, 4, 7, 8.*

RACQUETBALL

Why Racquet Sports Are Rated Tops as Whole Body Enhancers

Better to learn a few strokes than to live in danger of having one, and lack of exercise creates such a danger if you're over 30. A good way to reduce your risk of heart attack by 65% is to get a no-nonsense activity that burns 2,000 calories a week. And nothing burns calories and courts good health better than a court sport, if you are naturally fleet of foot, agile and have endurance (if you're not, cycling or running are better choices). Of the 13 sports America loves best and does most, the four that get top marks as whole body enhancers, says the President's Council on Physical Fitness and Sport, are running, handball, squash and tennis.

The President's Council on Physical Fitness Calls Racquet Sports Good Fat-Fighters

Three sets of tennis is the equivalent, in terms of overall cardiovascular benefits,[13] of 40 active minutes of football, one hour of roller skating, 60 minutes of volleyball or half an hour of rowing. If you don't own a rowboat, are too old for soccer, too slow for basketball and have a fear of merrily rolling along, that makes tennis twice as attractive—so does the fact that it burns an average of 400 calories an hour.

How Courting Fitness Can Improve Your Diet

It may even help shape up your menus. According to the Fitness in America Study sponsored by the Great Waters of France Corporation, 60% of all active tennis players claimed that taking up the sport had a strong, positive effect on their diet. Drawbacks? You need a court, equipment, a partner and fair weather and stick-to-it-iveness.

Why the Aerobic Institute Calls Racquet Sports "The Best Fitness in America"

Squash, handball and racquetball aren't for softies either. According to the National Squash Tennis Association, racquetball and squash are both

---

[13]What is your cardiovascular heart rate? Check it out—shooting above this so-called training rate can raise your blood pressure and tax your heart, undershooting it produces minimal fitness:
1. Subtract your age from 220.
2. Subtract your resting pulse.
3. Multiply by .6 (beginners) or .75 (moderately actives) or .85 (highly actives).
4. Add your resting pulse.
  Your training heart rate is _____.
  (Example: 220 minus 28 = 192. 192 minus a resting pulse of 70 = 122. 122 times .6 for beginners = 73. 73 plus 70 = 143—your training heart rate).

played inside boxlike rooms, using rackets to rebound a small hollow rubber ball in a duel of angles and strategy. Squash combines aerobic and anaerobic exercise. A match might take one or one and a half hours with very little rest between. A typical squash player runs and hits for half to three-quarters of the time on court. And what's true for squash is true of handball. It's not for the complete beginner.

Good Anti-Arthritis Activity

Both sports strengthen quads, hamstrings, buttocks, forearms and shoulder. Reaching for the ball in both sports increases flexibility and stretches shoulder and arm joints, making it good anti-arthritis activity. An hour can burn more than twice as many calories as tennis. The Aerobics Institute calls racquetball the best fitness activity in America.

The last but not the least benefit? Romance. According to Arizona State University psychologist Dr. Edward Sadalla, "Women find dominant men sexy and tennis players the sexiest of all."

If you're up to it—go for it. Have a complete physical first, then sign up for classes at the YMCA, the local racquet club or call your Parks and Recreation. Practice routines for partnerless players are detailed in any good racquet sport book.

And be sure to keep the eyes you have on the ball under wraps with proper peeper protection. Invest in a pair of strapped-on closed-eyeguards with lenses made of polycarbonate plastic (the same material used in bulletproof windows). It won't crack or splinter, says Canadian ophthalmologist Dr. Michael Easterbrook, a University of Toronto assistant professor, and protects you from eye injuries caused by speeding balls. Prices run about $40 or less. You can also get prescription lenses and have an optometrist or ophthalmologist shape the frame to fit your head.

And to be safer than safe, keep this number in your shorts pocket: (317) 926-1339 (for speedy sports medicine advice from the University of Indiana School of Medicine).
Longevity Benefits: *1, 2, 4, 6, 7, 8.*

WEIGHT TRAINING

According to Dr. Raymond Harris, President of the Center for the Study of Aging in Albany, exercise can retard some of the functional declines that accompany aging. Such as: loss of muscle mass, capacity for physical effort, flexibility, endurance, bone strength and efficiency of the heart and lungs. And according to Dr. Nila Kirkpatrick Covalt, writing in the *Southern Medical Journal* (July '81), "It even provides protection from one of the top 10 diseases of aging—arthritis. Exercise is one of the most beneficial therapies for this painful disorder."

Do you need weight training's number one benefit—more flexibility and upper torso strength? Here are two ways to test it out from the National Fitness Foundation:

1. *Upper Torso*

(Hang from a gym or parallel bar as long as possible)

Scoring (Minutes and Seconds)

Age	18–29	30–39	40–49	50–59	60 & over
Excellent					
Female	1:31+	1:21+	1:11+	1:01+	:51+
Male	2:01+	1:51+	1:35+	1:21+	1:11+
Very Good					
Female	:46–1:30	:40–1:20	:30–1:10	:30–1:00	:21–:50
Male	1:00–2:00	:60–1:50	:45–1:35	:35–1:20	:30–1:50
Good					
Female	to :45	to :39	to :29	to :29	to :20
Male	to :59	to :49	to :44	to :34	to: 29

2. *Stretch and Flexibility*

(Reach forward as far as possible while sitting—measure the inches from crotch to fingertips you can reach)

Age	18–29	30–39	40–49	50–59	60 & over
Excellent					
Female	23+	23+	22+	21+	21+
Male	22+	22+	21+	20+	20+
Very Good					
Female	17–22	17–22	15–21	14–20	14–20
Male	15–21	13–21	13–20	12–19	19–18
Good					
Female	to 16	to 16	to 14	to 13	to 13
Male	to 12	to 12	to 12	to 11	to 11

The Easy Exercise That Could Increase Your Strength 20 to 30% in Two Weeks

And one of the best of the exercises you have to choose from is working out with weights. According to Australian physician Dr. John Pearn, who put 50 untrained male college students through 20 minutes of workouts a day, all participants showed objective improvement in both absolute strength and pulse recovery times in the space of two weeks. The men's muscle strength increased by 20 to 30%, and their endurance (cardiovascular power) increased by 15 to 20%. Total exercise time over the two-week period came to only about six hours.

Weight Training Protects You from Heart Disease, Says the AMA

Weight lifting, in fact, is more than a muscle builder. Studies published in the *Journal of the American Medical Association* show that training with moderate weights and repeating the exercise many times improves levels of the kind of cholesterol that provide the most protection against heart disease. High-density lipoprotein (HDL) cholesterol, which transports cholesterol out of the blood increases while its counterpart, low-density lipoprotein (LDL) cholesterol, which promotes the uptake of cholesterol by arteries decreases when you work out with weights.

Special Ways Women Benefit

Weight work offers something special to the unfit female. Another *Journal of the American Medical Association* study of non-exercising, over-30 women who worked out on weight training machines three days a week for one hour all showed dramatic drops in blood fat after 16 weeks. Exercises that pull on the muscles are the ones that do the most to prevent or remedy varicose veins and osteoporosis, those two almost-for-women-only-after-50 disorders, advises Dr. Howard Baron of Manhattan's Cabrini Medical Center.

More Get-Up-and-Go than You Get from Jogging or Cycling

Besides building mid-life strength and endurance and lowering cholesterol, weight work with barbells and dumbbells (free weights) or machines (Nautilus, Universal, etc.) tones your muscles and tightens your body better than a more aerobic sport such as running and cycling. Although it isn't a top-flight weight reduction activity, it can burn 300–400 calories worth of fat an hour, off your top-heavy top or bottom—as much as an hour on the ice rink or the tennis court. (On the total fitness scale, weight work places third after swimming and cross-country skiing.)

Look Thinner in Eight Weeks

The next question is machines or free weights? Experts claim pumping iron can make the difference in the way you look and feel after four to six weeks of following a 40–60 minute routine three days a week. In eight to 12 weeks, in fact, you can significantly decrease the percentage of body fat and increase weight of muscle or lean body mass, says Steve Fleck, exercise physiologist at the University of Alabama at Birmingham. "You may not get a change in total body weight (unless you complement it with a diet) but you'll look thinner because you have less fat and more muscle."

Although both get you there, in general, machines tend to build up the lower body most effectively while free weights build the upper body—chest, shoulders, forearms and back.

How to Reduce Your Body's Three Hot Spots for Fat

Here are a few uplifting exercises to get you going on the body's three hot spots for fat:

To strengthen chest

- Lie on your back with your arms straight up in the air, a weight in each hand in an overhand grip (your palms facing the ceiling).
- Slowly lower the weights to your upper chest, just above the collarbone, keeping your elbows closer to your sides. Pause a moment, then push the weights straight up in the air again. Your arms should be perpendicular to the floor.
- Suggested starting weight: 5 to 8 pounds. Do two consecutive sets of six to eight reps and build to two sets of 12 reps.

To strengthen abdomen

- Stand comfortably, arms at your sides, a weight held in each hand in an overhand grip (your palms facing your sides).
- Bend to one side as far as you can, letting your hand with the weight in it slide down your leg as far as possible. Hold a moment, return to start, then bend to the other side.
- Suggested starting weight: Under 5 pounds. Start with 12 reps on each side; build to 24 on each side.

To strengthen lower back

- Stand with your feet comfortably apart, one weight held by both hands (use overhand or facing grip), your arms relaxed so that the weight is about at mid-thigh. Now bend over from the waist until the weight is resting on the floor, or is as close to the floor as you can manage.
- Come to a standing position, keeping your arms straight. Try to think of your hands and arms—and the weights—as dead weight to be raised only by the action of your body. Keep feet flat on the floor when you perform this exercise.
- Suggested starting weight: 9 to 10 pounds. Start with two consecutive sets of six to eight reps each, build to 12 reps.

Longevity Benefits: *4, 5, 8.*

MARTIAL ARTS/FENCING

Looking for a low-trauma aerobic activity (swimming and cycling are low-trauma; running, soccer and football are high-trauma)—a workout nobody else on your block is doing?[14] Try a martial art—or better yet, fencing. Neither one is the fancy-pants, sit-on-your-hands exercise it may seem. A vigorous workout such as karate, wushu or the oriental fist-and-weapon sport known as Shaolin, or a cat's-paws-and-calisthenics activity such as fencing or Tai Chi can add seven to 11 years to your life, if you've got an eat-right, sleep-well life to go with it, says the Women's Sports Federation.

Martial Arts offer you two things that mom-and-pop sports such as cycling don't—low injury risk and mental health. Because your weight is on the bike in cycling, not your body, according to the President's Council on Physical Fitness, there's a risk of shortening hamstring muscles, leg flexibility is reduced, you are exposed to traffic and air pollution, and most people pedal too slowly to derive maximum cardiovascular (heart/lung) benefit anyway. As the director of Boston's Wushu Institute puts it, "Calisthenics and aerobics are physically good but they are limited to the body and do very little for the mind."

The One Sport That Improves Your Mind as Well as Your Body

Take Tai Chi Ch'uan (pronounced Tye Gee Chwan) for example. This system of slow, continuous and rhythmic exercise (which may be on the menu at the local YMCA) is designed to maintain and improve physical and mental health with a minimum of bodily wear and tear. In one 15-minute routine, you do up to 108 soothing but muscle-developing movements. The system was developed voer 800 years ago in China and it's still being performed twice a day by millions of Orientals of all ages who consider it as much a part of their daily hygiene as brushing their teeth.

Why Martial Arts Produce Fitness Plus Tranquility

Martial arts activities exert a "tranquilizing" effect on the mind while simultaneously helping to regulate your blood circulation, keep your joints and muscle flexible and increase lung capacity, and they maintain the health of all body organs. Tai Chi exercise tones muscles, but unlike pull, push and punch calisthenics, the movements are slow and gliding, leading to a mind and body harmony, not agony, making this Oriental exercise a good choice for victims of lower back pain or arthritis or bursitis sufferers.

---

[14]What *is* everybody else on the block doing? According to the National Family Opinion, Inc., 85 million of us are busy bodies and the five sports we're busiest at are cycling, fishing, swimming, boating and jogging.

Burn as Many Calories as Jumping Rope

Karate and wushu, on the other hand, give you a more vigorous workout. Both systems of self defense are great ways to *stay* in shape if you are already half way there. A warmup followed by slapping, stretching and punching movements form the basic technique. An intense workout follows and this is followed in turn by a health-booster meditation break since the Chinese believe that the body can be healed by the mind when it is serene and focusing inward. Karate training promotes an awareness of the flow of Kn (energy) throughout the entire body. Briskly done, it burns as many calories as racquetball or brisk rope jumping sessions (600–700 per hour).

And although they are too slow-going (i.e., anaerobic) to get your heart pumping at the 60 or 70% of its maximum—the level required to produce what doctors call a measurable reduction in your heart risk—they're still anaerobic enough to promote a noticeable reduction of fat deposits in the body, if at a somewhat slower pace, fitness studies indicate.

What You Get from Fencing That Boosts Youthful Vigor

What's true for wushu or karate is true for fencing—with a few fringe benefits. According to the United States Fencing Association (USFA), fencing is a middle-range sport as far as calorie burnoff goes. It burns 12.9 calories per hour for every 2.2 pounds of body weight and it strengthens as it slims.

In a study conducted by Dr. Maurius P. Valsamis, manager of the U.S. Olympic Fencing Team in 1980, when lower-limb strength of a group of fencers was compared with that of athletes on professional hockey, basketball, football, soccer and lacrosse teams, the fencers were stronger than all the athletes except the football players. "No other sport conditions so totally," says Carla-Mae Richards, executive director of the USFA. "It helps legs, arms and breathing, and you can do it for the rest of your life."

Better yet, unlike running or figure skating, you can start later and still be a star. The better fencers start young, but the sport can be taken up at any age and played into the 80's.

Improve Your Brain-Power and Coordination

Like the martial arts, fencing improves the ability to make split-second decisions and it's as good as court sports such as tennis or racquetball for sharpening hand-eye and hand-foot coordination.

Getting in Touch

To find a martial arts course or class near you, call your nearest YMCA/YWCA or local parks and recreation department or write the following:

Tai Chi Association
Box 29344
Atlanta, Georgia 30329

Chinese Wushu Research Institute
247 Harrison Avenue
Boston, Massachusetts 02111
(info supplied on wushu, tai chi and shaolin)

To find the nearest fencing class, contact the United States Fencing Association, 1750 E. Boulder Street, Colorado Springs, Colorado 80909. **Longevity Benefits:** *5, 6, 9.*

YOGA

Would You Like to Know the Centuries-Old Secret of Lifelong Flexibility?

You're in celebrated company if you stand on your head. Yoga is the workout choice of Joel Gray, Helen Gurley Brown, Pauline Trigere, Alexis Smith and beauticians Vidal and Beverly Sassoon. No wonder!

"Yoga buffs," says Dr. Robert S. Brown, professor of psychiatry and education at the University of Virginia, "probably put a good price on longevity." With good reason. "Man is as young as his spine is supple" goes a yoga proverb. And no exercise gives you half the crack at flexibility that Hatha yoga does.

Four Benefits of Yoga That Slow Aging

What's the supple spine-extended youth connection? According to the Yoga Institute of America, a supple spine allows you to twist your body forward and backward, give it a lateral twist with ease, perform countless movements which improve the circulation, and tone the vital organs.

Yoga Provides a Key to Stress-Control and New Energy

Yoga's not a good way to lose weight or earn aerobic points, and it doesn't produce the "exercise highs" that result from increased levels of beta-endorphin hormones in your brain thanks to aerobics. But yoga does prevent atrophy of your dorsal and vertebral muscles, improves flow of blood around your spinal column, improves your posture, and helps prevent or alleviate arthritis or lower back pain. It even helps remedy fatigue because the fifth lumbar vertebra—that part of the spine upon which it is based—is positively affected.

Yoga also gets top marks for injury potential and tension reduction. And all you need is barefeet, a sense of fun and a bath tub and exercise mat.

To increase the benefits, follow up your yoga session with 10 minutes of running in place or a brisk walk or bike ride.

A yoga routine can be sensual as well as sensible. Here are two easy workouts to do in the water, three to do out of it and what benefits they have for you.[15]

Fill a clean tub with warm water, get in and get comfortable. Begin breathing deeply and regularly. Watch your body's reaction to what you are doing, bearing in mind that the best changes are gradual ones. Don't strain to do too much, especially if you have been inflexible for a long time. To get more benefits out of your holistic soak—use 1 to 4 pounds of Epsom salt. It helps to relax you by drawing cellular fluids up through the muscles to the surface of the skin. Another self-treatment is the "salt glow." Put sea salt on a wet wash-cloth and massage the skin. It couldn't hurt. Provide some ventilation around the tub.

End Lower Back Pain with These Two Exercises

The following two exercises free tension in the pelvis, massage the organs in the abdomen and release the lower back muscles:

Knee-to-chest wrap

• Lie back in the tub. Bring your knees to your chest.
• Breathe in as you hold your knees loosely with your hands.
• Breathe out as you gently squeeze your thighs against your belly.
• Repeat four times. Keep feet and ankles relaxed. As your thighs press your chest, you bring together the internal organs and push new blood and energy into them.

King of the waters pose (Also called the lion pose)

Sit up in the tub. Breathe in fully. At the moment of exhalation, try the following simultaneously:
• Open your mouth and your eyes wide. Stick out your tongue long and flat, making a sound like "Haaah . . . !" Imagine that your tongue reaches down beyond your chin.

• Stretch your hands and arms outward and slightly back, as far as they can reach.
• Arch your back.

---

[15]Exercise on an empty stomach and allow three to four hours after a full meal, one and a half hours after a small one and wait 30 minutes to eat after a workout.

Feel Better in 10 Ways with These Three Exercises On a Mat

The swan

(Helps eliminate back pain, minor sciatica, tension and fatigue; tones and strengthens the muscles of the arms, shoulders, back abdomen, buttocks and thighs.)

Starting position: Lie face down, legs straight and together, arms extended to sides at shoulder level.

Action: Count 1: Arch the back, bringing arms, chest and head up, and raising legs as high as possible. Count 2: Return to starting position.

The rocking horse

(Expands chest and firms chest muscles, relaxes the thoracic cage and improves breathing capacity.)

Start by lying prone; bend knees and reach back and grasp ankles firmly. Then, keeping arms straight, raise thighs three times. Don't pull up with arms. Instead, push feet out against hands. Rock. Repeat three to four times.

The peacock

(Increases suppleness and fluidity of movement in the spine, and develops strength in the muscles at the waist; corrects rounded shoulders, sunken chest and minor disc displacement.)

Starting position: Stand, feet shoulder-width apart, hands behind neck, fingers interlaced.

Action: Count 1: Bend trunk sideward to left as far as possible, keeping hands behind neck. Count 2: Return to starting position. Counts 3 and 4: Repeat to the right.

Want an even better alternative to flexing your way to fitness on your own? Call the local YMCA or nearest fitness center to find the nearest class.

Longevity Benefits: *5, 6, 9.*

5

501 Shortcuts
to a Longer Life

SHORTCUTS TO A LONGER LIFE

You don't have to use the long form for longevity in your daily life. There are a lot of everyday shortcuts that will get you there every bit as fast. Here are some of the best:

Eat Away the Years

Fat and sassy and you'd settle for sassy?

Eat fewer calories, substantially less fat of *all* kinds and take more vitamins, especially B-1, A and C. This is what did it for all the older women who looked younger and leaner in a 30-year study conducted by longevity researcher E. D. Schlenker and his teammates at Michigan State University.

Thigh anxiety?

Maybe you don't need to flatten those post-50 thighs. Maybe all you need is more PUFA, L-ornithine or L-arginine. The polyunsaturated fatty acids (PUFA) found in vegetable oils, lecithin and primrose oil supplements aid in the transportation of oxygen through the bloodstream, help maintain cellular health and regulate the thyroid gland which controls the burning of calories. What are L-ornithine and L-arginine? Two amino acids which supply a growth hormone that decreases as the body ages, often causing an elevated weight as a side effect. One out of every two people who supplement with these nutrients experience weight loss— often of 10 to 20 pounds by the end of two months. A good weight loss dosage is five or more 1 gram capsules a day.

Use safe herbs, not dangerous diuretics, if you have a few plus-50 pounds to lose

Best ones for appetite control and reduction of fluid retention (edema) are: chickweed, fennel seeds, burdock root, kelp, bladderwrack and chia seeds. Two more from your health food store that get the nod from the American Herb Trade Association: juniper berry and cornsilk.

Eat ethnic and lose weight?

You can do both if you choose wisely. Two diner's tips for dieters: Cantonese menus offer more foods with fewer calories than other types of Oriental cooking. The chopstick food that's most caloric? Sichuan/Hunan. Second least caloric? Almost anything Mandarin. A few calories to remember—bean curd soup, 39; egg drop soup, 94; ginger beef, 559; sweet and sour eggplant, 173; moo goo gai pan, 145; subgum lobster, 175; sweet and sour chicken, 1,163; braised shrimp, 448.

Watch out for imitation milk

This low-fat dry milk product is made primarily from whey and casein, two byproducts of cheese manufacture, but other ingredients include corn syrup solids for sweetness, coconut oil for richness, phosphates for buffering, mono- and diglycerides for emulsifying, carrageen or gums for thickening, artificial flavors and colors in some brands, and a variety of added vitamins and minerals.

It's cheap but it's not as nutritious as milk. It has only a third of the protein, two-thirds of the calcium and none of the magnesium in cow's milk. Worse, the coconut oil it contains raises blood cholesterol levels higher than real cholesterol in whole milk.

Sweet on sweets?

Here's how to keep dieting and cultivate a peaches-and-cream complexion for the lining of your stomach at the same time. Make peach butter. It's 50% lower in calories than jam, 60% lower in fat than butter and has less than 10% of jelly's sugar in each ounce.

Quick peach butter

• Place ½ cup almonds with ½ cup water in a blender; process until reduced to a liquid paste.

• Add 6 peeled, pitted peaches, ¼ cup honey or less and 2 teaspoons lemon juice.

• Process again until well-blended. Store, covered, in the refrigerator. 33 calories a tablespoon.

Variation: Substitute apricots or strawberries for peaches.

Tired of honey? Try aquamiele, a thick juice extracted from the heart of a tropical plant called *Agave atrovirens*. The juice was known to the Aztecs 2,000 years ago as "Food of the Gods." It's rich in natural sugars and contains only 20 calories per teaspoon. Available in jelly or tablet form from Botanical Products, Inc., 1093 S. Newcomb, Porterville, CA 93257.

Fat blood is blood with excessive cholesterol

It can lead to clogging of the coronary arteries and a heart attack, says the American Heart Association. And half of us over 40 have fat blood. The first line of defense, says the AHA, should be a cholesterol-lowering diet. Here's how to cut back on fat without forsaking cheese: 1 ounce of Camembert cheese has as much saturated fat (8 grams) as a serving of fast-food chili. Just as tasty? Well-fermented tempeh, the soybean protein substitute for meat and cheese.

Two easy ways to lower your salt intake and never know the difference?

Beat a path away from your local burger heaven and switch to Angostura's bitters. Bitters are better than salt because this tasty liquid seasoning invented 150 years ago, and used largely in mixed drinks, contains only .16 mg. of sodium per teaspoon (salt has 2,325 mg.) and makes a zippy flavor-enhancer in everything from vegetable soup to fruit desserts. Another good ultra-low-sodium salt substitute? Tabasco sauce.

What do one cup of rue, broccoli, spinach or corn and 20 french fries have in common?

They all supply 4 to 8 grams of fat-free protein—roughly 10% of your RDA. Have a broccoli-spinach rice-and-carrot casserole with corn chips on the side, for example, and you're 20 grams of protein to the good, so hold that high-protein whopper on the back burner.

What do such meatless eats provide?

Vitamins A, B-1 and C, plus iron and calcium—the five nutrients Americans between 25 and 40 are most deficient in, say food consumption surveys by the USDA. To "healthify" your diet, eat larger amounts of fresh fruit, vegetables and whole grains. And think twice about that raise. It could be hazardous to your health. "The more money Americans earn, the less time they spend preparing meals at home, so the more fat they eat," warns the Agriculture Department. Fat is considered a major factor in stress-related ills such as cardiovascular disease, ulcers and cancer.

It's green, it's a cinch to grow and it has only 13 calories and almost *0* sodium and supplies your RDA for A, C and anti-fatigue folic acid—it's parsley

But don't use it in sprigs. Here's a super-calorie-cheap way to put more of it in your diet: *Low-Sodium Parsley Potato Boats*: Stir ¼ cup fresh chopped parsley into ½ cup plain yogurt. Add one squirt lemon or lime juice, fresh pepper and spoon over two hot baked potato halves.

Why are there fewer cases of hardening of the arteries in China, Greece, Russia and India than the United States?

"Because," says professor Hans Reuter of Cologne, Germany, "they eat lots of cholesterol-reducing garlic." Another good way to shape up your cardiovascular system? Try groaning. "Groaning can be healthy," says Dr. Louis M. Savary, co-founder of Inner Development Associates. "It lowers tension and releases anxiety, and produces vibrations within the body which effect a kind of inner message. To avoid embarrassment? Groan alone. You can't relax and groan efficiently when you're afraid someone is listening," says Savary.

Reduce Caffeine—Increase Your Energy

The caffeine in coffee is good for getting you going but the lift doesn't last. Caffeine saps energy. According to Dr. John Greden, former director of psychiatric research at Walter Reed Army Hospital, in susceptible people even a few sips of coffee will elevate blood sugar levels, and heart rate and blood pressure increases. Capacity for muscular work may be temporarily stimulated, but since these effects are accompanied by nervousness and irritability, you haven't really gained, you've lost.

Two ways to improve your body's adrenalin reserves and oxygen intake without sugar or caffeine? Juice and cookies. One glass of apple juice contains the adrenalin-boosting power of 5 teaspoons of table sugar; and the whole-wheat flour, nuts, wheat germ and oils in a good baked goodie are all sources of oxygen-improving vitamin E, says the USDA.

Caffeine abstinence is the only known cure outside of surgery for fibrocystitis, the breast lump disorder that can lead to cancer for older women. If even decaf isn't enough of a caffeine cutback for you but you love the taste, here are a few foods that provide satisfaction substitutes—

1. *Dandelion and Chicory*: The powdered root of both of these uncommonly healthy common weeds make great no-kidding-it's-not-coffee substitutes. And both can be blended in various proportions to suit your taste. As a treat, sweeten the way American Indians did—with natural maple sugar or a piece of honeycomb.

2. *Sunflower Seeds*: Buy sunflower seeds in the shell. Roast until brown

in a slow 300° oven. Grind in a coffee or nut mill to a fine powder. To prepare, steep as for tea. Proportion: 1 tablespoon powder per cup.

3. If what you really miss most is not coffee but *coffee ice cream*, get the flavor by sprinkling decaffeinated espresso powder over plain vanilla.

4. If your holiday cup of cheer is without caffeine and you'd like to do it without fat as well, skip Half-and-Half and light cream. Both have twice the saturated fat (2 grams per serving) of this healthy high-calcium home-made creamer. *No-Fat Coffee Cream*: Put one-half cup of skim milk powder, 1 cup of liquid skim milk and 2 tablespoons of safflower or peanut oil into the blender and liquefy. Makes one cup.

5. Coffee drinking increases stomach acid and sets the stage for periodontal disease and osteoporosis because it blocks the uptake of calcium. Three tasty alternatives: Spanish chestnuts, chickpeas, carrot root. All provide an alternative cup of cheer, advises the New York Botanical Garden. As a bonus, these nut and vegetable beans won't hook you the way caffeine in the coffee bean does. All must be oven-roasted till coffee-colored, then ground and perked.

6. What's not coffee but could be and comes caffeine-free from a *Dahlia root?* Dacopa instant, sold in packets, 4 calories a cup. Good iced. Not on the shelf? Write Dacopa Foods, P.O. Box 139, Manteca, CA 95336.

7. *Dried corn* may beat decaf. A cup of corn coffee is rich in brain-perk carbohydrates so it improves your alertness but helps you leave those caffeine-created-high times behind. Roast kernels of whole dried corn in a 200° oven until deep brown. Put through a coffee grinder or grain mill or crush with a heavy rolling pin. Boil, perk or drip to desired strength. Sweeten, lighten and sip. For "Instant Corn Coffee," scatter a thin layer of cornmeal on a cookie sheet and bake at 300° until it darkens. Use 1 tablespoon a cup.

8. Roasted malted barley is not only a natural sweetener, it makes a milder-flavored-than-decaf cup of coffee and gives you non-dairy calcium, too. Look for it in two instant coffee substitutes sold at supermarkets—Celestial Seasoning's Breakaway blend, Orange Cappuccino. Or buy a whole barley brew to perk from scratch such as Wilson's Heritage at your health food store.

* * * *

Love cappuccino? Carob, a sweet powder derived from the pod of a tropical bean, gives you the taste without the unhealthy caffeine.

Copycat Cappuccino

Combine:

One 2 oz. jar freeze-dried decaffeinated coffee powder, plus ¼ cup carob powder

½ teaspoon ground cinnamon (or mace)

Optional: 2 to 4 tablespoons whole milk powder may be added for a richer flavor and more calcium.

• Stir ingredients well. Store in a tightly covered container. Makes 1 cup decaffeinated cappuccino.
    • Use 1 rounded teaspoon of mix in a cup. Add boiling water and stir.

* * * *

Strong tea can be strong stuff. Here's the punch three favorites pack:

• *Green teas* (green gunpowder and jasmine): 2 to 7% the caffeine of coffee.
• *China teas* (Earl Grey, black currant, China oolong): 10 to 20% of the caffeine of coffee.
• *Breakfast and Indian teas* (English and Irish breakfast and Assam): 30 to 35% of the caffeine of coffee.

Stay Healthy by Staying Happy

Don't be afraid to cry, and listen to more music

A good bawl and good music beats stress, suggests Dr. Margaret Crepeau of the Psychiatric Nursing Center at Marquette University School of Nursing in Milwaukee. "People who cry freely suffer less inflammation of the large intestines." In her study of 128 men and women, she found that "Crying reduces our susceptibility to stress-related diseases . . . The more crying a person does, the less likely he is to suffer from such diseases." She adds that, women cry a significant five times more often than men, on the average. "If we don't cry, our health suffers." If you can't cry, a little Bach may be just as good. According to alternative medical expert Dr. David Bresler, "Music has been shown to accelerate body metabolism, muscular activity and respiration. It influences pulse rate, blood pressure and minimizes the effects of stress . . . Music may even break down cholesterol in the bloodstream."

Put on a happy face with music

"Music is energy, just like food," says California psychologist Dr. Steve Halpern. "Having the right music around the house is as important as having the right food and the right vitamins." If it's sweet enough, it can even lower your blood pressure, kill pain. "Music is an extremely powerful tool," says Nancy Hunt, a St. Louis, Missouri music therapist. "It has a direct physiological effect on people. It increases blood volume, decreases and helps stabilize heart rate and lowers blood pressure . . . makes us relax . . . even have good feelings."

Looking for a Mr. Right who tips the scale?

According to British research specialist Dr. Anthony Harris, who has concluded a 10-year study of 2,500 couples of various weights, the attraction rate between fat men and fat women is 7.7 on a scale of one to 10. There is almost eight times the attraction rate between a muscular man and a muscular woman, and twice the attraction rate between a fat man and a slim woman. The happiest marriages of all were found between both thin and fat women and mates similarly shaped. They also had the lowest divorce rate. Happily married and neither fat nor thin? You probably see yourself as others do. "Most people think they're fat when they really are not," says Los Angeles nutritionist Dr. Robert H. Brooke. "While over 50 percent believe they're overweight, only 22% actually are."

Amino acids lift the spirits

According to longevity researcher Dr. Roy Walford, *a shortage of amino acids such as methionine found in aging brains, contributes to premature senility.* "Amino acids (which are the building blocks of protein) minimize the effects of oxidation which weakens immunity and DNA repair. Another lift-the-spirits amino acid Walford swears by is cysteine in 300 mg. tablets. If you're not a pill popper, three top food sources of both acids are eggs, soybeans and sea vegetables such as kelp. Goofing off is good for a have-a-happy-day-outlook too. "People think better when they lie down," concludes a new Columbia University study. A horizontal position with the feet slightly raised enabled subjects to solve math problems. 7.4% faster and with 14% greater accuracy than they could on their feet.

Happiness is a diet that keeps you slim and disease-free

How much do you know about what you eat? Test your smarts. True or False? 1) The FDA allows some 80 chemicals as ingredients in the making of peanut butter and wine; 2) Riboflavin is also known as The Glucose Tolerance Factor; 3) 150,000 hip fractures each year are caused by jogging and osteoporosis; 4) A 3-ounce serving of broiled chicken has 560 calories. *Answers:* 1) False. Wine only; 2) False. It's called Vitamin B-2; 3) False. Osteoporosis is the cause—jogging is the prevention; 4) False. It has 115.

Feeling down in the mouth?

Take a walk. We need sunlight to feel happy, says Dr. William Fry, who is the clinical associate professor of psychiatry at Stanford University. What happens if you're a closet case? Your body produces high levels of a hormone called melatonin which causes depression. Victims of severe depression can often be cheered up by opening curtains, shades and blinds, even adding artificial light. Better yet, advises Dr. Normal Rosenthal of the National Institute of Mental Health (NIMH), "take a walk in the sunshine whether it's winter, summer, fall or autumn."

Get Moving to Fight Aging

Be physically active

Stay physically active, says gerontologist Dr. Alexander Leaf, professor of Clinical Medicine at Harvard Medical School. "This is the one major difference I discovered between what people 100 years and older are doing compared to our country." (Best all-around long-life activity? Swimming.)

Fifty-plus and stressed?

Put yourself in motion or get a paintbrush. Exercise can reduce stress by as much as 80%, according to a recent year-long, computerized study of exercise conducted on executives and professionals working under constant stress. Men who followed the varied exercise program had an average 43% drop in anxiety. The highest drop was 80%. Those in the exercise group also emerged happier and more pleased with themselves. If a little locomotion doesn't relax you, change your environment. According to the *Brain/Mind Bulletin*, different colors set off a chain reaction of hormonal secretions, and each has a distinct effect upon the adrenal glands. Pink, for instance, sends a message to the adrenals telling them to slow down. "This reduces blood pressure, slows the heart rate and relaxes muscles. It is very difficult to express anger while being exposed to the color pink," notes the *Bulletin*. Stress-arousing shades include yellow, orange and red.

According to Dr. William Kannel, medical director of the Framingham Heart Study in Framingham, Massachusetts, "At least 16 million Americans over 35 are physically inactive. People in the sedentary group have a coronary death rate of about 7%. But those in the active groups have a coronary death rate of about 4 to 4½% . . . Even a modest amount of activity can be beneficial . . ." Here are four short workouts: (1) Jump with both feet, twisting the whole body from side to side the way skiers do when descending a mountain. Then bend knees deeply. (One minute.); (2) Kick one leg to side, then to the front, eight times each. Switch to other leg and do the same. Now hop as you kick, eight times each. Repeat. (One minute.); (3) Jog in place; lean forward slightly. (Four minutes.); (4) Combine all three of these steps to music. (Four minutes.) Walk around after these vigorous exercises until you cool down and your breathing slows.

Three heart-healthy good deeds

Learn to take your own pulse; take a class in something aerobic to raise it, such as cross-country skiing, squash and running up and down stairs, and eat at a restaurant where the foods are low-fat.

How to take your pulse: Find your carotid artery with the tips of your fingers in the front strip of muscle that runs vertically in your neck. Take your pulse rate just after exercising by feeling and counting for 10 seconds. Multiply by six. If your heart rate was 15 for 10 seconds, your target exercise heart rate is 120. The lower your exercise pulse is, the stronger your heart. If you've done your daily dozen and you'd like to do your heart one more good turn, add a few drops of hawthorn oil to your diet. It's a medicinal herb that aids circulation, strengthens the pulse beat and regulates heart rhythms without side effects. Ask your health food store for tincture of hawthorne berry. Write the New York Heart Association, 205 East 42nd Street, New York, N.Y. 10017 for a guide to heart-healthy restaurant meals. (Enclose a self-addressed, long business envelope with two 22-cent stamps.)

Hate to work out?

Head for the hills. Living in high altitudes above sea level seems to reduce oxygen tension, and this has the same effect on increased exercise, helping to prevent heart disease. If living on high doesn't improve your heart's health, church-going could. According to Wake Forest University psychiatrist Dr. Richard Proctor, "The greater your conviction and the greater your belief in God, the more likely you are to be healthy of mind and body." Faith, says Proctor, promotes peace of mind and reduces the chances of suffering stress-related illnesses, especially heart disease.

It's better to be caught napping than hanging if you're looking for a new post-40 health perk

Hanging from the ceiling upside down wearing gravity inversion boots can harm your back and send your blood pressure through the roof, say osteopaths. So-called "inversion boots" which are used daily by tens of thousands of health-seekers appear to be dangerous if you have heart trouble, spine ailments or glaucoma. Blood pressure greatly increases after three minutes or more of suspension.

How's your stay-young exercise IQ?

True or False:

1. You can't over-exercise. The more you do, the better.
2. Physical exercise relieves mental stress.

3. Pain can be relieved by strenuous sustained exercise.

Answers:

1. False. Over-training leads to injuries.
2. True. Activity releases endorphins in the brain that have a tranquilizing effect.
3. True. Euphoria resulting from strenuous exercise often blocks pain.

What good deeds can a good jog do for your diet?

According to the *Fitness in America* study conducted by Perrier Bottling Company, runners eat 30% more vegetables than the moderately sports-active individuals, and 35% more than "low actives." Runners also eat 79% less junk food and 5% less cola, and take 30% more vitamin and mineral supplements. And of all the groups surveyed, runners reported the lowest use of antacids, aspirin and tranquilizers.

Whatever you do decide to get physical at, make sure it isn't something you've got an inherited pain potential for

According to Robert Nirschl, an orthopedic surgeon and director of the Virginia Sportsmedicine Institute in Arlington, if your parents suffer from back pains or foot problems, you may be vulnerable, too. Consider sports that don't strain those parts of the body. And dress all your parts properly. "Wearing vinyl, rubber or plastic garb while doing strenuous exercise can be fatal," warns Dr. Leon Rottmann, a human development specialist with the University of Nebraska. "It knocks the body's thermostat out of kilter and prevents natural body cooling by sweat evaporation." Rottmann cites the case of a 21-year-old who died of a heat stroke while running in a vinyl sauna suit. What's best? Cotton.

Don't run with radio headphones

Running may be what keeps the cardiologist away, but it could be what brings the otolaryngologist running if you're wired for sound when you jog. "Permanent hearing loss can result from frequent use of portable headphone cassette players and radios even if the volume is not particularly loud," says hearing health (otolaryngology) authority Dr. Craig Senders, assistant professor at the University of California Medical Center at Davis. At the University of Iowa in Iowa City, volunteers listening to headset stereo for only three hours a day at moderate volumes experienced some hearing loss with "very noticeable" impairment in some cases. The good news? Hearing normally returns to normal in 24 hours after the headsets are removed and if the hearing loss is detected in time, it can be reversed.

Give your hands a health workout

Here's a massage recommended by sports physician Dr. Phillip Lee of the University of Iowa: Spread baby oil (or mineral oil) over one hand. Do the following exercises slowly to each hand: Grasp the back of the oiled hand at its widest point (the base of the pinky and thumb) and squeeze. Release, then spread your oiled fingers wide. Do 10 times; turn your oiled hand palm side up, and with the knuckles of your other hand, knead the palm two minutes; grasp and gently pull down the length of each oiled finger to a count of eight; with arm outstretched, make a fist. Move only the wrist, curling fist toward the inner forearm. Relax.

How to Stay Young by Looking Good

Doing the cube?

Not to worry, says Temple University dermatologist Ray J. Yu. Sugar may be no treat for your teeth but it's sweet stuff for plus-30 complexion because the glycolic acid in sugar cane helps keep skin smooth by balancing the skin's acid-alkaline moisture levels.

Out of apples? Raid the fridge. Lemons and oranges also have the Big Mac's moisturizing potential. But don't shower. Soap and water remove dewy do-good acids from the skin.

And don't count on fruit as a substitute toothbrush. According to the Rochester, New York Eastman Dental Center, "Eating an apple is not a good rinsing-the-mouth way of ridding the mouth of foods such as bread or candy. Rinsing with water is better."

Reduce your blood pressure and treat yourself to a younger body

There are 14 factors that make you feel and look older than you are, according to the Gerontology Research Institute of UCLA. The three that add two or three years are blood pressure over 140/90, overweight and smoking over 15 cigarettes a day. The two factors that make you look and feel at least two years younger are blood pressure under 130/75 and no history of chronic diseases.

Coffee lips?

Switch to herb tea. Coffee's caffeine destroys vitamin A, and vitamin A deficiency is a major cause of dry, cracked lips. "If you find yourself always using balm because your lips feel dry, you're caught in a cycle," says Dr. Robert Tietschel, a dermatology professor at Emory University in Atlanta, Georgia. "This dependency creates an artificial micro-climate and causes lips to forget how to adapt to climate changes. RX? Kick the chapstick habit. "It takes about 30 days for lip tissue to readjust to the real climate."

And for appearance, reduce caffeine and boost your intake of such vitamin A foods as spinach (2,230 I.U.), endive (825 I.U.) and wheat grass tablets.

Owl-eyed? It can make you look older

Try sniffing extracts of these herbs to beat insomnia, suggests the International Fragrance Foundation: basil, camomile, lavender, melissa, mandarine, orange, meroli, rosemary, thyme or rose. Simply add a few drops of the oil of your choice to a warm bath or vaporizer, or massage directly into skin. As a bonus, these fragrant oils, available from herb suppliers and health food stores, can correct minor skin balances such as oiliness and dryness, and skin disorders such as acne, psoriasis and eczema.

How's your tyrosinase level?

If it's high and you're Irish, your "beauty-puss" potential may be on the line. Lots of the enzyme tyrosinase, says the Skin Care Institute of America, increases production of the pigment that causes tanning and "it's highly active only in certain areas of the skin in people of Celtic origin (Irish, Scottish)." Result? Freckles. There's no known way to fake out freckles except to stay inside. But while you're there, there is something you *can* do to lick chapped lips, advises Lawrence E. Lamb, M.D., Professor of Medicine at Baylor College of Medicine in San Antonio. Don't lick them; rub with mineral oil, Vaseline, lanolin or propolis lotion; get more fluids in your diet and step up your vitamin E and A intake.

On the go? Don't let your beauty diet lose its bloom

One deli Reuben or Big Mac with fries has twice the calories (800) of a three-piece Italian manicotti dinner (under 500). Forbidden eats in flight can be worse. Five ounces of Eastern Airlines Chicken Kiev is 600 calories, and a single slice of TWA's chocolate cake has 200. A teaspoon of sugar added to every cup of hotel coffee means 18 more calories. Three times a day means 39,240 calories a traveler's year—an annual addition of 10 pounds. Cut back on sweets.

Don't use petroleum-based hair products

If you care for your hair, the safest thing you can run through it besides your fingers isn't isobutane chloride, propane or glycerol—it's wheat bran. Isobutane and propane are petroleum-based ingredients used in popular hair lubricants and gels that ignite easily, say researchers at Johns Hopkins Medical Institute's Burn Center. Petrolatum products including petroleum oil and jelly, propane, isobutane and methylene chloride, are three times more flammable than hair greases containing water, lanolin and glycerol. Here's how to make your own *60-Second No-Frills Shampoo*: Combine ½ cup wheat bran with 1 tablespoon baking soda. Rub into hair and brush out thoroughly to remove dirt and oil.

Looking good? Just make sure what you're using's good for your looks

Test your bodycare I.Q. True or false?

1. All of the following are emollients—ingredients that smooth, soften or moisturize the skin: a) aloe vera; b) lanolin; c) sweet almond oil; d) honey.

2. Government regulations on the manufacture of bodycare products are strictest for products to be used on which area of the body? a) mouth; b) eyes; c) scalp; d) underarms.

3. Which of the following because of its effects on bodily functions is designated as a "drug" by the FDA? a) deodorants; b) shampoos; c) skin creams.

4. The skin care ingredient most likely to cause a rash is: a) coloring; b) preservatives; c)fragrance; d) emulsifier.

Answers:

1. True

2. b)

3. All three (according to the law, any product promoted as being useful in diagnosing, treating or preventing disease . . . or affects the structure or function of the body may be designated a drug).

4. c) (How to spot an offender? Rub a small amount of the product on the inside of your elbow. If it produces any redness, don't buy it.)

If you want to fight aging better, keep track of reps and laps while you're counting calories

Besides getting slimmer, you'll wind up with better skin. According to Dr. Albert M. Kligman, professor of dermatology at the University of Pennsylvania School of Medicine, who has been documenting the dermatological effects of exercise by using three-dimensional photographs to measure the number, depth, width and distribution of wrinkles in the face, women who exercise regularly have fewer wrinkles than those who don't. One reason? Exercise thickens the skin and that improves wrinkle-resistance. If that doesn't motivate you, a similar study by the Exercise Physiology Department at the University of California, San Diego, probably will. According to study director Dr. James White, bags under the eyes of a group of sedentary middle-aged women disappeared only weeks after the group began a trampoline program. Three sports with good skin conditioning effects are swimming, roller skating and aerobic dancing.

Like to look younger longer? Eat less and sleep more

"Beauty sleep is an accurate concept. Insufficient sleep reduces circulation and contracts the capillaries causing dehydration and sagging and causes dark circles under the eyes by reducing collagen in the tissues," says insomnia expert Dr. Samuel Dunkell. When you're not snoozing, lowering the boom on calories can make you look 10 years younger. Dr. Charles Barrows of the National Institute on Aging, who did it with animals on a diet slashed to 60% of its usual caloric intake, says it works with humans, too, and as a bonus, you'll probably live 33% longer. Don't want to cut back? Fasting one day in three may produce the same beauty effects.

Thirty-year-old skin at 50?

A cinch if you increase your body's supply of NAPCA, a sodium salt that decreases in the skin after 40. The more NAPCA you get, the fewer wrinkles you'll see. NAPCA is produced in the body by L-glutamine. Good sources include amino acid supplements, soybeans and low-fat yogurt.

What goes into your toothpaste could be age-you-faster additives

Mildly abrasive commercial brands contain 53.85% dicalcium phosphate dihydrate, an abrasive; 43% sorbitol-water mixture, a sweetener; 1.5% sodium carboxymethyl-cellulose, an emulsifier; 1.5% sodium lauryl sulfate, a wetting agent; 0.1% saccharin, another sweetener and 0.05% methylparaben, a preservative. Go to your health food store for brands free of these.

Another way to prevent decay besides brushing? More natural light. Studies indicate that insufficient daylight increases the tendency to develop cavities five-fold, while natural daylight improves resistance to tooth decay, even on a high-sugar diet.

Quick Remedies for Feeling Better

Give guar a chance if you're serious about lowering cholesterol

Studies of patients who have taken cholesterol-reducing drugs for more than two years without success, showed a typical blood cholesterol level reduction of 11% when 5 grams of the food additive *guar gum* was taken three times a day with meals. Guar (or xanthan gum or powdered guar) is sold at most health food stores or by mail from Now Foods, Villa

Park, Illinois 60181. It can be baked into bread or used as an addition to juices, soups or casseroles, even sprouted.

Headache? Your security blanket could be to blame

Trying to catch a few extra winks in the morning by pulling bed covers over your head "turtle-fashion" to block out light is a headache-maker because it reduces the flow of oxygen to the brain. And if you're older, grayer and allergic to boot, watch out for such pain-maker foods as milk, cheese, eggs, chocolate, tea, wheat, orange and apples. Migraine sufferers studied by Dr. Jean Munro of the National Hospital for Nervous Diseases in London, England, had an average of three of these in their diet. Simply eliminating them brought relief in less than two weeks.

Having nyctalopia?

Maybe it's because you're deficient in rhodopsin. And both conditions may be the result of Xerophthalmia. Xerophthalmia is old-fashioned vitamin A deficiency which causes the common complaint you might call night blindness and ophthalmologists call nyctalopia. Making sure your vitamin A is normal (5,000 I.U.'s daily) should solve everything by increasing the rhodopsin you need to see after dark. This is a protein in the retina behind the eye, says Dr. Carl F. Gruning, O.D., that is used up each time your eye is exposed to bright lights.

Another better-vision trick is eye exercise 10 minutes a day. Two optic exercises are used widely by millions of spectacle-free citizens in China, which relax the focusing muscles of the eyes and increases blood circulation, says Dr. Bradley Straatsma, an ophthalmologist and director of the Jules Stein Eye Institute at UCLA School of Medicine.

Here's how—keep eyes closed, keep fingernails short and hands clean. Sit with elbows resting on a table and repeat each exercise six to eight times a day.

Exercise 1: Place thumbs on lower jaw and index and middle fingers against both sides of nose near nostrils. Lower the middle fingers and massage with index fingers.

Exercise 2: Use the thumb and index finger to massage the nose bridge. Press downward, then upward.

If you *don't* run, *do* get more omega-3 fatty acids in your blood and lessen the risk of coronary thrombosis

Eskimo and Japanese fishermen who consume large amounts of fish oil and fatty fish have the lowest incidence of heart disease in the world. Omega-3 fats are richest in trout, haddock, salmon, mackerel and sardines, and are also available as a food supplement (look for the words EPA or DHA on the label). Three grams a day taken with meals is a good heart-protective dose, says the American Medical Association.

Don't reach for a new-fangled drug, reach for old-fashioned baking soda

Bicarb seems to counteract lactic acid buildup in the muscles and keeps you going longer, says Dr. Robert Fitts, director of the Exercise Physiology Lab at Marquette University in Wisconsin. High levels of lactic acid in the muscle tissue caused by hearty exercise is a common cause of fatigue. Besides adding a little baking soda, it helps to reduce the acid-forming foods such as wheat, meat and dried fruits in your diet and concentrate on more alkaline foods such as leafy greens, root vegetables and sunflower seeds.

Is your health playing dead? Maybe what you need is a super bulb, not a super supplement

Duro-Lite and Vita-Lite are specially coated, low-glare fluorescent light bulbs designed to give off low levels of ultraviolet light unlike ordinary bulbs that distort light and aim primarily for brightness. Used by the University of Massachusetts, the American Ballet Theatre and NASA, the new light which is sold at health food stores, is said to switch off fatigue, improve eyesight and even nourish the skin. Or have a good laugh. According to recent studies at the University of Maryland, laughter can relieve the pain of arthritis and may even have an impact on hypertension. The key is improved circulation. A good laugh also aids digestion by stimulating enzyme secretions; it even acts as a gentle laxative. Pediatricians say babies start laughing at around 10 weeks, and by four years children are laughing once every four minutes. It is estimated that adults in really good health laugh hundreds of times a day.

Healthy herbs that prevent exercise burnout?

Try red sage, a remedy for players' asthma, coughs, colds, bronchitis, fevers of all kinds and sore throats. You name it. Sage works on the lymphatic system, moving toxic material out of the body, cleanses an overworked liver, heals the nerves and is a good tonic in a tea cup for fitness headaches. If sage leaves anything to be desired, your ace in the hole may be quassia, which Utah herbalist Lucy Hart calls "an excellent tonic to tone up a rundown system." A bonus for the bend-an-elbow-prone jock? Quassia even removes the appetite for alcohol. Quassia and red sage teas are sold at health food stores.

On the go and you've got the runs, don't despair and don't take drugs

Here are four ways to get revenge on Montezuma's revenge that are healthier than prescribed apothecaries:

- *Arsenicum 30X*: A not-so-side-effect remedy available from homeopathic pharmacies (every town has one). Two tablets after each loose stool does the trick.
- *Activated Charcoal Tablets*: Two or three every eight hours.
- *Papaya-Leaf Tea*: In any amount.
- *Liquid Chlorophyll*: One to two teaspoons every hour.

And add two acidophilus tablets between meals. Non-toxic, pure stabilized oxygen drops also help you cope with "tourista." At your pharmacy or from Life Quality Products of Stockton, California.

Down in the mouth because you've filled your fill-your-mouth quota for the day?

Try "aroma therapy." According to Daniele Ryman, author of *The Aromatherapy Handbook* (Century Publishing), "Body organs or glands which are in a state of depression selectively take up different essential oils and use them in the same way they would utilize vitamins and minerals in order to function properly." Fragrances that work best to fight diet blues are angelica, basil, carrot, lemon, coriander, ginger eucalyptus, lavender, mandarin, marjoram, melissa, mint, and parsley.

Music and pain suppression

Sweet music has pain-suppressant potential, according to John Kabat-Zinn, Ph.D., director of stress-reduction and relaxation at the University of Massachusetts Medical Center. "Music takes the mind to another place, reduces your awareness of pain and puts your psyche someplace else for awhile, in a place where there is no pain—psychic or physical." Why does it work? One theory is that some kinds of music can produce in the brain the same "feel good" chemicals that running and meditation produce called endorphins, natural opiates secreted by the hypothalamus, which reduce pain's impact. Best bets if you're going to soundproof your health and put a smile on your face? Anything Baroque by Handel or Telemann, Beethoven's "Fifth Symphony," anything by Bach, especially the "Mass in B Minor" and Dvorak's "New World Symphony."

Confucius (circa 500 B.C.) recommended the consumption by everyone of a little ginger every day, to insure health and longevity

The Greeks praised ginger as a general tonic. Culpepper prescribed it to help digestion, warm the stomach, clear the sight, expel the wind and heat the joints. Inhaled like snuff, dried ginger induces sneezing. Chewed, it increases the flow of saliva. In the stomach it stimulates digestion; in the bloodstream it dilates the blood vessels. And there's nothing that soothes a sore throat like ginger boiled in water that is sweetened with honey.

Tobacco—good and bad

Lighting up may be bad for the heart, but it's just what the doctor ordered for today's tennis elbow and tomorrow's heartburn. Tobacco juice, says Dr. Rulon S. Francis, head of the Human Performance Research Center at Brigham Young University in Provo, Utah, heals bruises 20% faster than most other existing treatments. Trainers often treat player's injuries with tobacco poultices. And according to Dr. Shuh-Ji of the University of Kentucky, the protein in tobacco leaves can be beaten to a fluff like egg white, and is more complex and efficient in its amino acid makeup than milk or meat. Tobacco leaf protein has also been used for relief of kidney disease and digestive ailments.

If your gums are bleeding, maybe you need a change of climate and a change of fruit

According to Dr. John Manhold, a professor of general and oral pathology at the University of Medicine and Dentistry of New Jersey, gum disorders are a sign that stress may be interfering with your body's natural healing process—or even causing some tissues to break down. Even if you can't get away, you can get more stress-reductive vitamin C into your diet. It's as close as your next fruit smoothie. Just make sure the fruits are apples and oranges, not oranges and bananas. According to a study conducted by the Department of Nutrition, Ministry and Health in Jerusalem, Israel, fruit mixtures consisting of fresh orange juice, apple and banana showed a 75 to 80% decline in total vitamin C content when banana was added.

How to Live Longer by Loving Better

Who's likeliest to be the longest-lived person on the block?

According to the Director of Baltimore's Gerontology Research Center, married women who are financially secure, highly intelligent, sexually active, with three children and long-lived ancestors, as a class enjoy the longest lifespans in America.

Don't overlook good buddies if you're looking for longevity

According to psychologist James J. Lynch, Ph.D., "Social contact has a demonstrable effect on brain size. Young rats deprived of their pals can lose up to 10% of their brain size. And if you put old rats—the equivalent of a 65-year-old person—in with young rats, the old rats' brains grow . . . The brain has this ability to keep reshaping itself."

Short on friends?

Get a dog. "Talking to pets can reduce your blood pressure," says Dr. Aaron Katcher, associate professor of psychiatry at the University of Pennsylvania. "Talking to and touching animals is stress reducing." Studies indicate that pet-owner patients hospitalized for heart attacks had higher survival rates than non-pet-owners.

Want to fight fat, fatigue and funk?

Socialize. After studying the ages and socialization habits of 7,000 people, Dr. Lisa Berkman of the University of California at Berkeley, concluded that people who take an active role in socialization are more likely to live longer. People who stay at home alone are more likely to be overweight, drink too much alcohol and smoke cigarettes than the socially active.

Take a friend to lunch or help the handicapped

The life you lengthen may be your own. The divorced, widowed and elderly die soonest from heart disease. Loneliness is the number-one cause of premature death today, says James Lynch, Ph.D., of the University of Maryland School of Medicine. Why is being a lonely-only a killer? Because it's a stresser. Stress causes hypertension and coronary heart disease as well as suppressing the immune system, the body's first line of defense against disease, says psychiatrist George Vaillant M.D., of Harvard University.

Fatigue-fighter—oyster powder

"Oyster powder is very helpful in beating all forms of fatigue, including sexual," says French nutritionist expert Dr. Robert Mason, president of the College of Natural Medicines in Paris. "Oyster powder has almost the same chemical composition as milk—another famous, all-around anti-fatigue food." What makes the lowly mollusk a better pick-me-up than "moo" juice? Twelve oysters, shells and all supply 200 times more iodine and as much protein as 3½ ounces of red meat. Oyster shell powder is sold in U.S. health food stores as a calcium supplement, or by mail from Now Foods, Villa Park, Illinois 60181.

Like to be sexier and smarter by adding only one good food to your life-extension diet and dropping one life-shortening bad habit?

Eat more wheat germ, a top-rated source of the mineral zinc, says mineral researcher Dr. Paul Eck, and give up that bad deed weed. Chronic cigarette smoking is synonymous with low energy. "That's why smokers need a cigarette after sex. Both smoking and sexual activity use up zinc and sex uses zinc-linked stores of energy. A cigarette stimulates the glands producing a temporary energy boost," says Eck. The zinc and thinking link? "A hippo-campus, causing confusion and dullness," says *Clinical Psychiatry News*. "A reduced coping capacity" may mean you are low in zinc. Healthy zinc levels decrease irritability, nervousness and restlessness, and, according to Irving Leopold, M.D., sometimes improve the I.Q. by as much as 20 points in less than 12 months. Best sources besides wheat germ are raw nuts, seeds, sprouts and oysters.

Happiness is good health and your pinkies are a perfect indication of whether you're in the pink of it or not

According to Dr. Edward Kowaleski, Professor and Chairman of Family Medicine at the University of Maryland School of Medicine in Baltimore, fingertips that turn white at the slightest temperature change may be a tipoff you suffer from Raynaud's disease, a condition causing impaired circulation, especially in the hands and feet, while a flushed hand, showing too *much* circulation, could indicate polycythemia vera, another circulatory disease. "Pale nails often indicate blood loss or anemia. Spoon-shaped and nails that are paper-thin and fragile may spell thyroid or calcium problems," says Kowaleski. What's a tipoff your hands are up-to-snuff? "Normal blood vessels would appear light blue, look soft and smooth, not pulsating. Anything else," says Dr. Kowaleski, "could indicate a disorder in the cardiovascular-renal (heart and kidney) system." Two foods for healthy hands and heart? Vitamin E-rich wheat germ and magnesium-rich raw nuts.

6

Sources of Help
for Staying Young

GADGETS THAT HELP YOU PROLONG YOUR LIFE

Does good health after 30 need a gadget to keep it going? No, but a good one—such as a blood pressure monitor—can be a life saver—as well as a life-extender.

Here are 16 that are tops. Available by mail (M), major department stores (D), sporting good stores (S), and/or quality health pharmacies (P).

1. Exercise Weights

• Handheld (1 to 20 lbs.); $20 and up.
• Travel weights (average weight 2–5 lbs.); under $40—can be adjusted.
• Lace weights and ankle weights; about $20.

Recommendations: All three increase aerobic conditioning benefits and calorie burnoff. But if you're going to buy, just invest in one. They can be used equally well for running, walking, dancing, etc.

Sources: S, D, M.

2. Blood Pressure Monitor

Look for a model that is lightweight with a digital display of blood pressure and pulse. A good buy for hypertension sufferers.

Recommendations: The Timex Health Check has them all; about $70.

Sources: M, P, D.

3. Portable Gym

For doing strength exercises and aerobics in small quarters. A must if you travel a lot.

Recommendations: Life Line; about $35.
Sources: S, D, M.

4. Food Computer

Foolproof way to prevent cheating for here-we-go-again weight-watchers. Computes the weight, calories, protein, fat, sodium, carbohydrates, cholesterol, etc. of more than 500 foods.

Recommendations: The Compucal; about $130.
Sources: M, P.

5. Test Your Salt Intake Kit

Good gadget for anyone on a doctor-prescribed low-sodium diet. Special strips are dipped into the first urine voided in the morning. The chloride part of salt in the urine reacts with chemicals on the Saltex strip to darken the bottom end. The larger the area that turns dark, the higher your previous day's salt intake.

Recommendations: The Saltex "qualitative chloride titrative strip" is considered almost as accurate as laboratory salt tests.
Sources: P, M.

6. Skin Calipers

A good companion to the bathroom scale for weight-watchers. Consumer's version of the calipers doctors use to measure body fat percentages.

Recommendations: Fat-o-Meter; $10.
Sources: from catalogs, S, P, M.

7. Medical History Pendant/Card

Worn around the neck, the pendant carries your medical history plus doctor's and emergency phone number on microfilm. Details visible when held to a light under a magnifier.

Recommendations: A good one sold by Mediscope, 101 Fifth Avenue, New York, N.Y. 10003; $14.95 plus $1.50 postage. A variation is the medical history card—a microfilm reproduction of your medical history (an EKG, tracing, optional) along with its own magnifying glass from National Health and Safety Awareness Center, Suite 1625A, 333 No. Michigan Avenue, Chicago, Illinois 60601.

8. Vitamin C Test Kit

One drop of a test solution on the tongue measures your tissue levels and absorption rate of ascorbic acid. Available from ABROCA, Inc., Box 5529, Maple Street Station, Beverly Hills, California 90210; about $10.

9. Plaque Detection System

A must if you have an advanced case of periodontal gum disease. Developed by a dentist, a special solution makes invisible plaque on your teeth glow yellow so you know where to clean and when you've done the job.
Recommendations: Clairol's Plak-Chek; under $15.
Sources: P, M, D.

10. Electronic Bath Scale

Displays your weight to the nearest half pound more faithfully than old-fashioned models in easy-to-read digitals.
Recommendations: Health-o-Meter; a good buy under $40.
Sources: P, M, D.

11. Exercise Bikes

If you can't or won't cycle outdoors, a good buy. Plan on paying a minimum of $200 for this all in one way to workout your heart/lungs/legs/ lower torso. Ergo-cycle types let you vary pedal speed and adjust your workload.
Recommendations: The Body Guard; about $400.
Sources: D, S, M.

12. Air Ionizer

This tabletop gadget for the allergic, the sleepless and the stressed to plug in, drags smoke, dirt, dust, pollen virus, odors, bacteria out of the air and recharges the air with improve-your-mood negative ions.
Recommendations: The tabletop ionizer from Consumer Health Products, 23251 Collins Street, Woodland Hills, California 91367; about $90.
Sources: M, P.

13. Vision Screening Test

A better way to spend a buck to prevent blindness. This 10-minute test spots muscular degeneration, a leading cause of blindness after 50, detects poor vision, other eye diseases. Also checks distance and close-up vision and degeneration caused by blood vessel damage. Available from the National Society to Prevent Blindness, 79 Madison Avenue, New York, N.Y. 10016.

14. Emergency Dental Kit

Dentist-designed quick fixes for toothaches, broken tooth, loose or lost bridge, filling or crown, cracked denture. A must for travelers.
Recommendations: The ED kit from Dental Alternatives, 3141 Ann Street, Baldwin, New York 11510.
Sources: P. M.

15. Food Dehydrator

Make your dried fruits and vegetables, even dry your own eggs and milk at a nutrient-preserving 120°F or below. Increases the vitamin, mineral, enzyme and fiber levels in food. $40 and up.

Recommendations: The best units have adjustable thermostats and run close to $200. The Harvest Maid Dehydrator available through the Sears, Roebuck catalogue (400 East Fordham Road in the Bronx [212/938-1200] or at 137-61 Northern Boulevard in Flushing, Queens 718/445-9050, Catalog Item 11G5134C; $100).

16. Sprouter

To simplify the efficient sprouting of a variety of different seeds. These gadgets range from $10 and up.

Recommendations: To grow up to 30 different kinds of seeds all at once, you need the sprouting system from: Spruton, Inc., 1285 Collier Road, N.W., Atlanta, Georgia 30318.

MAIL ORDER SOURCES

- The Sharper Image   Medical self care devices. Catalog
  406 Jackston St.   available.
  San Francisco, California 94111
  (800) 344-4444
- Edmund Scientific   Medical self-care devices. Catalog
  101 E. Gloucester Pike   available.
  Barrington, New Jersey 08007
- Wysong Health and Fitness Corp   Medical self-care devices. Catalog
  4925 No. Jefferson Ave.   available.
  Midland, Michigan 48640

FOOD AND SUPPLEMENT SOURCES[1]

If your local market or health food store does not have it, write away. Catalogs available.

Source

Aphrodesia   1, 2, 3
282 Bleecker Street
New York, N.Y. 10014

---

[1] 1 = fresh and dried herbs, spices and seeds, powdered dairy products
2 = vitamins and herbal supplements
3 = special health foods and exotic foods
4 = cookware kitchen gadgets

Now Foods 721 N. Yale Villa Park, Illinois 60181	1, 2, 3, 4
Walnut Acres Penns Creek, Pennsylvania 17862	1, 2, 3, 4
Indiana Botanic Gardens Box 5 Hammond, Indiana 46325	1, 2, 4
Herb Gathering 5742 Kenwood Kansas City, Missouri 64110	1
Wysong Health and Fitness Corp. 4925 No. Jefferson Avenue Midland, Michigan 48640	1, 2, 3, 4
Brookstone 127 Vose Farm Road Peterborough, New Hampshire 03458	3, 4
Vermont Maple Box 53 Jericho Center, Vermont	Pure maple syrup, maple sprinkles (dried syrup granules), natural gums and candies.
Robledo Import and Export 4297 S. W. 75th Avenue Miami, Florida 33155	100% pure whole cane sugar (Labeled *Panelista*).
Santaroni Rockefeller Box 1349 New York, N.Y. 10185	Brazilian herb tea (rejuvenation tea).
Crayon Yard Corp. 75 Daggett Street New Haven, Connecticut 06519	Sunpot yogurt-maker and cultured food cooker.
Sprout Letter Publications Box 62 Ashland, Oregon 97520	Sprouting supplies, food supplements, books, T-shirts, juicers and more.
New England Cheesemaking Supply Co. P.O. Box 85 Ashfield, Massachusetts 01330	Cheese- and yogurt-making suppliers; wine and vinegar kits; cookware

GETTING HELP IN STAYING YOUNG

National Organizations	Services
Dr. Denham Harmon American Aging Association University of Nebraska Medical Center Omaha, Nebraska 68105 (402) 541-4000	Research
Mrs. E. Henderson, Director American Geriatrics Society 10 Columbus Circle New York, N.Y. 10019 (212) 582-1333	Research; no special service for non-members
Richard A. Passwater, M.D. Chief of Research American Gerontological Research Laboratories 529 Southview Avenue Silver Springs, Maryland 20904	Research
Dr. Bernard L. Strehler Association for the Advancement of Aging Research University of Southern California 2025 Zonal Los Angeles, California 90007 (213) 746-6019	Research
National Council on Aging (NCOA) 1828 L Street N.W. Washington, D.C. 20036 (202) 223-6250	Fee-free information; request details
National Senior Sports Association 317 Cameron Street Alexandria, Virginia 22314 (703) 549-6711	Conducts regional and national tours in numerous sports
National Geriatrics Society 212 W. Wisconsin Avenue Milwaukee, Wisconsin 53200 (414) 272-4130	Pamphlet and newsletter available.

National Institute on Aging (NIA)
Information Office
Building 31
Bethesda, Maryland 20205

Many public services;
books, pamphlets, films
and cassettes available at
low cost. Write for catalog.

National Institute of Mental
Health (NIMH)
Section of Mental Health of the
Aging
5600 Fishers Lane
Rockville, Maryland 20852

Many public services;
books, pamphlets, films
and cassettes, available at
low cost. Write for catalog.

Gray Panthers
Retired Professional Action Group
(sponsored by Ralph Nader's
Public Citizen)
3700 Chestnut Street
Philadelphia, Pennsylvania 19104

Pamphlet and newsletter
available. Write for details.

American Association of Retired
Persons
1225 Connecticut Avenue N.W.
Washington, D.C. 20036

Request publications list.

National Chairperson
Task Force on Older Women
% NOW
1957 East 73rd Street
Chicago, Illinois 60649

Request publications list.

National Health Federation
5001 Seminary Road, #1330
Alexandria, Virginia 23211
(703) 379-0589

Consumer advocate health
group. Write for
membership details.

Center for Science in the Public
Interest
1501 16th Street N.W.
Washington, D.C. 20036
(202) 332-9110

Consumer advocate health
group; newsletter, posters,
books and more. Write for
membership details.

Cinemercia
9477 Brighton Way
Beverly Hills, California 90210

Around-the-clock,
nationwide program on
longer-life medicare and
more.

Association for Holistic Health
Box 9532
San Diego, California 92159

Pamphlets and newsletter
available.

Linus Pauling Institute of Science and Medicine 2700 Sand Hill Road Menlo Park, California 94025	Publications on vitamin C and cancer and other disorders of aging.
Association for Medical Health Alternatives and Clearinghouse Box 112 Clearwater, Florida 33511	Pamphlets and newsletter available.
National Cancer Foundation, Inc. 1 Park Avenue New York, N.Y. 10016	Fee-free information; request list.
American Heart Association 44 East 23rd Street New York, N.Y. 10010	Fee-free information; request list.
Arthritis Foundation 1212 Avenue of the Americas New York, N.Y. 10036	Fee-free information; request list.
American Diabetes Association 18 East 48th Street New York, N.Y. 10017	Fee-free information; request list.
National Parkinson Foundation 1501 N.W. Ninth Avenue Miami, Florida 33136 (305) 547-6666	Pamphlets available.
Parkinson's Disease Foundation William Black Medical Research Bldg. 650 West 168th Street New York, N.Y. 10032 (212) 923-4700	Pamphlets available.
United Parkinson Foundation 360 West Superior Street Chicago, Illinois 60610 (312) 664-2344	Pamphlets available.
National Center on Black Aged 1424 K Street, N.W., Suite 500 Washington, D.C. 20005	Pamphlets available.
National Indian Council on Aging P.O. Box 2088 Albuquerque, New Mexico 87103	Research on longer life pertaining to minority groups.

"To succeed, consult three old people," goes a Chinese proverb. Better yet where health is concerned get in touch with an organization that makes youth-keeping its business. You might consider a health ranch, rejuvenation farm or longevity spa (the 1985 tag for rejuvenation was $375–$2,500 per week) to help you get the stay younger upper hand on your personal renewal program.

Here are some good accredited choices in each category:

Rejuvenation Clinics/Resorts[2]/Ranches/Spas/Private Specialists

The Golden Door
P.O. Box 1567
Escondido, California 92025
(619) 744-5777

The Greenhouse
P.O. Box 1144
Arlington, Texas 76010
(817) 640-4000

The Kerr House
Grand Rapids, Ohio 43522

Rancho La Puerta
Tecate, California 92080
(619) 478-5341

Canyon Ranch Spa
8600 Rockcliff Road
Tucson, Arizona 85715
(800) 742-9000

New Age Health Farm
Neversink, New York 12765
(914) 985-2221

Yoga Vacations
Box 255
Helena, Montana 59624
(406) 442-5138
Sea Pines Behavioral Institute
Sea Pines Resort
Hilton Head Island, S.C. 29928
(803) 671-6181

---

[2]*Note*: To check out a resort's credentials before you check in, write or call the Better Business Bureau in the state of location.

New Life Health Spa
Lifeline Lodge
Stratton Mount, Vermont 05155
(802) 297-2600

Villa Vegetariania Health Resort
Box 1228
Cuernavaca, Mexico
3-10-44 (telephone)

Dr. Benjamin S. Frank
7 East 80th Street
New York, N.Y. 10021
(212) 988-7800

Longevity Hotlines (toll free)	*Services*
Tel-Med	Taped medical library explaining causes and cures of age-related ills. Check your local directory for telephone number.
Second Surgical Opinion Hot Line (U.S Dept. of Health and Human Services)	Guide to specialists in your area for non-emergency surgery, call (800) 638-6833
Association of Heart Patients	Heart disease, pacemakers, more, call (800) 241-6993. Georgia residence call (404) 523-0826.
Diabetes Foundation International	Brochures and referrals, call (800) 223-1138. In New York State, call (212) 889-7575.
Cancer Hot Line (National Cancer Institute)	(800) 525-3777

Index